TRAVELS OF A DOCTOR
A MEDICAL DRIVE THROUGH THE EU

DR. GERALD MICHAEL

TRAVELS OF A DOCTOR
A MEDICAL DRIVE THROUGH THE EU

Matador
9 De Montfort Mews
Leicester LE1 7FW, UK
Tel: (+44) 116 255 9311 / 9312
Email: books@troubador.co.uk
Web: www.troubador.co.uk/matador

ISBN 978-1848760-271

Typeset in 11.5pt Bembo by Troubador Publishing Ltd, Leicester, UK

Matador is an imprint of Troubador Publishing Ltd

To my family

Contents

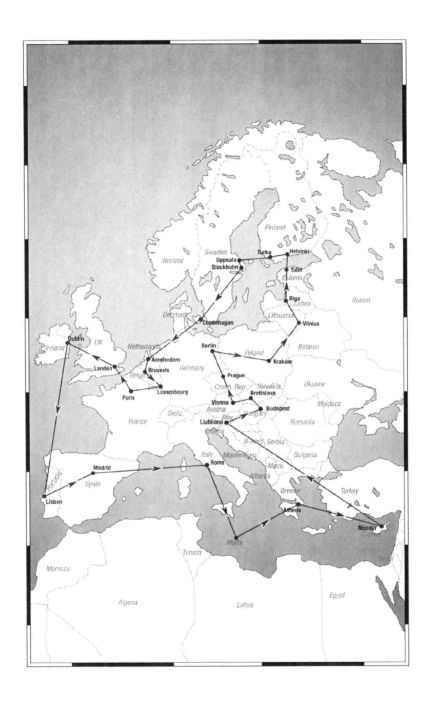

Map of route

Introduction

Who is involved?

Well firstly of course I am. I was born in 1936 and qualified as a doctor in 1960. I became a GP in North West London in 1963 and have been in the same practice ever since. When I joined I was the younger of two partners, and when I retired as a partner in 2006 I was the oldest of seven.

My father and grandfather were GPs but the line stops there because my children have chosen other careers. I married Wendy in 1962 and have two daughters Lucy and Victoria. I have also a son, Jeremy, who with his wife is a very experienced world wide traveller and gave me lots of advice, but had no direct role in this project so does not come in to the story again. I have four nephews, the third being called Rod. The lady in my satellite navigation system is called Gladys. Wendy, I believe, does not like her as she says, remembering Princess Diana's words, that "three in a marriage is rather crowded"

How it all started

At the beginning of 2005 I realized I was going to be seventy in June of the following year and it was time to think about retiring at least from the responsibilities of being a partner.

I have many hobbies but one of my favourites is travel, and Wendy and I go away several times a year, as going abroad, even for a day, has the same thrill for me as when my father drove my mother, sister and me to Switzerland in 1947. The idea of fly-drive to the south of France or Italy is absurd to me. Just getting into my car is a thrill and the two days spent getting down to the Mediterranean coast, stopping for good meals and a nice hotel, is an essential part of the holiday.

I probably enjoy all methods of journeying equally and any article in the paper on cars, ships, roads, planes or trains attracts my attention. I have a nice car and enjoy driving it. It has all the modern giblets including air-conditioning, sat-nav and adaptive cruise control. This last is a sort of extra cruise control which automatically causes the car to slow down to the same speed as the vehicle in front.

I thought therefore I could combine this love with something useful so I planned a journey to start the week after I retired. The intention was to drive, using ferries where necessary, to every country in the European Union and interview an English-speaking GP, find out about the health system in his country and report back.

My friends and family thought the idea crazy and somehow this spurred me on. Wendy was encouraging, mainly I think because she thought it would be dangerous for me to go alone and also I believe she became caught up in the excitement of the idea. She went home for six days in the middle and my nephew Rod joined me in Istanbul – yes I know Istanbul is not in the EU - but when you see the problems in going to Cyprus you will understand. Wendy's first break was when we were in Istanbul, when she flew home on the plane which brought out Rod. Rod stayed with me and shared the driving until we got to Budapest and then he returned home and Wendy came back. Rod was with me for one of the more difficult stretches driving through Turkey, Bulgaria, Romania, Serbia and Slovenia. Apart from this last, which is in the EU, all the other stops involving him were for one night only so he did not have time to relax. However he seems to have had a good holiday and like me he enjoys arguing and this passed the time very agreeably. I remember that the ethics of free-range versus battery chicken farming took up many hours.

Wendy went home for a long weekend in Stockholm where for the only time I was on my own and, after seeing a doctor in Uppsala,

I did the comparatively short two day drive to Copenhagen, where I retrieved her from the airport.

I missed my family and friends over the three months but Victoria flew out for a day to join us at Bratislava and of course I ran up an enormous phone bill. We hoped to save money by using a device in my computer called Skype but found it disappointing. Different friends came out to spend a day or two here and there, one couple coming with us from Vilnius to Riga and another joined us in Rome and again in Brussels at either end of the trip. Four friends came to see us in Berlin.

The planning was the hardest part, especially finding the doctors and sorting out Cyprus, more of which later, but the car problems, ferries and hotels all took time. In fact, the route was over more than twelve thousand miles and involved booking where possible and going on fourteen ferries.

After I started the planning I could never remember whether the idea of the trip came first followed by the idea of interviewing the doctors as a rationalisation for it, or whether it was the other way round. Anyway as time passed, both the travel and professional element absorbed me equally.

What I wanted to discover

The main aim was to do qualitative research into general practice. Most research is quantitative where double blind trials are done. In these trials one group of patients is given the drug under test and another dummy tablets which look similar. Neither the patients nor, until after the trial is completed, the doctors know which group is which. The size of samples is usually large and statistical tests are done to determine how large they need to be for the trial to give reliable results. Qualitative research is different. Clearly there cannot be large figures in this sort of audit as each interview took about two hours. Also, obviously, there was no blinding in that everyone involved knew who was who. The objective, therefore, of this work was to discover how general practice worked in each country.

3

I thought long and hard about what I wanted to find out about general practice in Europe and I prepared a questionnaire which I used as a guide. As a general practitioner, I am trained to ask open questions of patients, inviting them to answer in their own way. As this is the only method of interview I know, I used the questionnaire as an aide-memoire, not as a detailed tick box instrument. Although, as in general practice, this has a great advantage of ease of communication, it meant that necessarily some questions were missed, although all the main gist of the doctor's world was included.

After discussing it with colleagues, I amended it several times and while actually on the journey, experience led me to make further changes.

I was painfully aware that I would be mostly seeing only one doctor in each country and as far as possible I had to get him (or of course her) to describe to me the working conditions for the whole of his nation. Obviously his view may not be representative so my findings are no more than an impression. Fortunately the doctors seemed to understand what I wanted and I had the feeling that they tried to base their thoughts on the whole of their system.

My only interest is what we call primary care, which is mainly general practice but occasionally I mention other services. I was mostly interested in the equivalent of our National Health Service although, as we shall see, private practice looms much larger in some countries. Although most countries have a subsidised system of providing health care to their citizens, it is not necessarily through a government funded scheme such as in the UK. Sometimes it is organised, albeit on a compulsory basis, by insurance companies, others by the local community like the town council, and in Greece by the trade unions. To make the writing simpler I shall usually refer to the system or the state or even the national health, but I will always mean the same thing by these terms.

I asked each doctor about the number of doctors and patients they had in their practice and I was often shown round the premises. I wanted to know what sort of staff such as nurses, secretaries and receptionists they employed and if they worked alone or in a whole team including other professionals.

4

Access is a very sore issue in this country so obviously I inquired how easy it was for patients to get an appointment and how long these lasted. Also I wanted to know if they were available to offer phone consultations. Were the face-to-face consultations interrupted by phone calls? What arrangements were offered to their patients in evenings, nights and weekends? Were home visits still done?

I needed to know about the money issue both from patients' and doctors' perspective. Did patients have to pay anything towards the cost of the consultation and if so how much? We are so used to this being free over here we could, without knowing, expect this in all the EU but this would be a mistake. Then as a doctor myself I wanted to discover how my European colleagues were paid. There was a wide variety of answers to these questions.

I asked about the ease and methods of referring patients to specialists. (Mostly I use the terms specialists and consultants interchangeably.) I tested a few examples such as how long it would take to see a skin specialist and how long it would take for a patient to get a hip replacement after referral.

The management of medical records is a very important part of British general practice for several reasons. As well as forming a life-long history of every person's illnesses, including investigation results and treatment, they also form a snapshot picture of how well a doctor or a practice is doing at any one time in managing a particular illness such as high blood pressure or diabetes. We also find that keeping accurate contemporary notes helps us defend ourselves if ever there is a complaint. It was important for me therefore to explore the systems used elsewhere.

When I read a novel I get upset if the author suddenly implies that some character is eventually going to come to a sticky end; and I prefer not to know until the time comes. However I cannot resist saying at this point, and I hope that it does not spoil the story for you, that I found the issue of the differences of record keeping between British and other European doctors, when allied to a notion of 'ownership' of patients, one of the most important philosophical themes of this work.

We discussed how doctors went about treating illness and usually got on to treating common long term diseases such as high blood pressure and diabetes, but several others as well. In the bad old days, each doctor was a law unto himself and treated illnesses in his own way, and his method might be quite different from anyone else's. It was rather similar to gardening, where old Adam knows what is best using lots of experience but not necessarily any real knowledge. Well, in the fifties and sixties, doctors learnt to study scientific double blind trials we came across earlier and our treatment became more rational and of course more similar to each other. Later specialists in academic royal colleges and specialist medical societies such as the British Hypertension Society or The British Thoracic Society and many others developed guidelines for the best treatment of their illnesses and many doctors adopt these.

In the last few years there has been the Scottish Intercollegiate Guidelines Network (SIGN) which started in 1993 and gives excellent guidelines on the management of most illnesses, and The National Institute for Health and Clinical Excellence (NICE), which is a government body set up to advise on the best treatment for illness with an additional cost effective remit. So it can be seen we are well served with advice and information in this country. Most British GPs, sometimes a whole group, as in my practice, others as individuals, even if they work in groups, have developed guidelines from these national ones. Most of us see this as an enormous advance on what went on in the past but a few regret the loss of individuality and even loss of freedom. I thought it important to explore these issues with doctors in the rest of Europe.

Although we have few restrictions on what we can prescribe in this country this is not necessarily the case elsewhere, so this was an issue I discussed. Other topics included internet access, certificates, alternative medicine and health promotion.

Training is an important issue. This included how doctors were trained for general practice and what facilities they had for keeping up to date afterwards. Were they forced to continue learning and did they have any form of appraisal? In the UK it has been impressed on us to take notice of poorly performing doctors and take action to protect their patients as well as themselves. I asked about this issue and also about any complaints they had, or risk, of being sued.

Finally, after I started the journey I found that in not all countries did GPs do the same range of work as us, so I included questions about it as I went along.

For those of you who are interested I have appended a copy of my last used questionnaire aide-memoire at the end.

Planning – Finding the doctors

I thought finding the doctors would be easy but this took more time than anything else. The difficulty of making the contacts and the behaviour of the doctors caused more trouble than I expected. The Royal College of GPs (RCGP) publishes an annual rather like the Beano of my youth. Until a few years ago this had a page of members who worked abroad. This included their contact details and I assumed the college would send me the list and I could phone each one. However, since the Data Protection Act, this is not allowed. Anyway, they were helpful and agreed that if I drafted an email to the doctors setting out what it was all about they would pass it on to all their European members. This produced about six replies most of which have been useful. These contacts have been reliable, returned emails promptly and sounded interested. Two were so kind that they invited us to stay with them.

The draft email is as follows

Dear Dr

I am a GP practising in North West London. To celebrate my retirement next summer I intend to drive to all 25 EU capitals using ferries when necessary to find out about general practice in the rest of Europe. The level of practice I am looking at is the local health system in place that would cover an ordinary worker and his family in your country. I am not looking at private practice unless that is the usual system for workers. Also I am not looking at practice in place only for people with social security issues. This is meant to be a qualitative

7

survey. I will stay in each city at least 2 nights and 3 if the intervening day is a Sunday. On the intervening day I would like to meet you for some time to learn about your work.

The three headings I will be exploring are firstly, what are the problems of general practice in your country? For example, how easy is it for patients to get to see you and how long can you spend with them? Is it quick and easy to refer to secondary care and what are relationships like with local specialists? Are you able to maintain continuity of care?

Secondly, what arrangements are in place for continuing medical education? Are you required or encouraged to have any form of personal development plan? Do you have any form of appraisal? Thirdly, I am interested to know what the standard of life is for a GP in your country. What are GPs' premises like? (I would appreciate it if you would show me yours.) Do you have to be on duty out of hours? From the point of view of pay do you know how your standard of living compares with the UK?

I know that amongst my own colleagues their personal answers would be different from each other even in my own locality so I will ask you about your personal knowledge of other GPs' experiences that you know of.

These are preliminary ideas which I will refine during the next year.

I would be very grateful if you would be kind enough to let me know if you could see me. My address is (XXXX) and my email address is (XXXX). If you would prefer not to let me have your details please reply to (A named secretary)at the **RCGP.**

My trip will start in Dublin at the end of June going anti clockwise through Europe. For example I will be in Nicosia at the end of July and Warsaw mid August, Scandinavia at the end of August and followed by the Benelux countries and finishing in Paris early September.

Best wishes

Gerald Michael

Then I tried WONCA - no don't ask - well actually it stands for World Organisation of Family Doctors and I know this does not fit but it is not my fault. They have a European branch and their UK representative, when I emailed him, made it quite clear that as I was not an academic and had done no previous research he could not even ask WONCA to help. I had in fact done a project which had been published in the *British Medical Journal* (a peer reviewed publication), but this was more than twenty years ago and I did not think he would be interested. I then tried the colleges of general practices in each country starting with their web site. I usually found a secretary who told me to send an email and she would pass it on to a doctor. In about half the cases this worked but with the others there was no reply after a few phone calls and emails. One doctor sent me a rather suspicious email virtually asking me what business I had wasting the time of an important academic like her.

Dear colleague,

I forwarded your mail to the head of the general practice department of our university in Vienna, but obviously nobody replied.

My practice is not in the city.

I was not so sure if your mail is a serious one (I am suspicious concerning internet/mails – usually even don't open unknown mails)

I would have expected more details on how you chose my address, who gave you the idea to this project, is there any organisation backing it, are you in contact with any of the known GP/family physician organisations of WONCA?

Your plans and wishes do sound a little bit peculiar to me, - I am sorry. For instance: how come you already know dates from August ??

Many of your questions have been answered in previous surveys, or are available at Health authorities.

Good luck

I replied with more information and she sent a very warm and apologetic reply and has been happy to agree to see me and has also arranged meetings with a colleague in another town.

Next I just tried surfing the web putting in "English speaking primary care doctors" and naming the town. The only contacts that came from this were some names on the American Embassy sites. They did not lead me very far as I could find only specialists or private clinics. At this stage I was hoping to stay within state health systems. Then I tried phoning the best hotel in town and asking the concierge for the name and phone number of the doctors he sent ill guests to. This worked a treat but there were problems. The doctors being in the private sector were, as is the wont of private doctors, usually charming and agreeable but after the first contact there was often no further return of phone calls or emails. Where I was successful I realized that a private doctor would not be representative of the national system. One doctor understood this and took the trouble to pass my details on to a more suitable doctor who agreed to see me. Painfully slowly the list built up. I remembered having been invited to a patient's wedding to a doctor who had trained in Europe. I contacted him and he gave the name of a delightful doctor in his country. My nephew, Rod, has a friend who lives in Europe and his neighbour is a GP, and he agreed to see me.

Finally I got back to the RCGP and they told me they could send me details of WONCA members through the post but not electronically; apparently that makes it legal with the Data Protection Act. This has been most satisfactory. A personal email mentioning how I got their name has worked in all the remaining countries and these were the sort of doctors I needed.

I was passed round a chain of doctors in Cyprus until the most helpful one discovered that none of his colleagues could see me without permission from the Cypriot Ministry of Health. I wrote to them twice and they gave me their blessing by sending me a formal letter of approval and fixed me up with an English speaking GP in Nicosia:

REPUBLIC 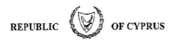 **OF CYPRUS**

REF. Nr: M.P.H.S. 5.31.004
TEL. Nr: + 357 22400233
FAX Nr: + 357 22305352

MINISTRY OF HEALTH
MEDICAL AND PUBLIC HEALTH SERVICES
1449, NICOSIA, CYPRUS

Dr Gerald Michael
23 Tretawn Park
Mill Hill
London
NW7 4PS

27 March 2006

DRAFT LETTER

Re: Visit of Dr Gerald Michael to a General Practice setting in Cyprus on Friday the 21st of July 2006 for the purposes of a survey

I am authorised to inform you that special arrangements have been made so that you can meet a GP on Friday the 21 July 2006, for the purposes of your survey. The details of the Health Center are the following:

Aglandjia Health Center,

86, Kyrenia street, 2113, Plati, Aglandjia- Nicosia, Cyprus.

Dr in charge: Dr Elli Angelidou

Tel.: +357 22 305240

Fax: +357 22 305253

Please feel free to contact me again for any further information.

Dr. Evi Missouri,
On behalf of Acting Director
Of Medical and Public
Health Services

Cc: Dr Elli Angelidou, Aglandjia Health Center, 86, Kyrenia street, 2113, Plati, Aglandjia- Nicosia, Cyprus

EM/..

11

When the list was almost complete the weight of what I was planning became easier and I could start looking forward to the holiday.

Planning the route

Not only have I always been passionately fond of travel but I have always liked collecting lists. I have a long list of foreign countries I have been to and another list of their capitals I have visited. For no sensible reason I try to keep the latter nearly as long as the former. This is often at considerable inconvenience and I missed Canberra but managed Ottawa and Pretoria. I had already been to twenty-one of the EU countries and also all their capitals. When planning the route I realized that Cyprus is now a member and somehow I would have to go there. The journey involved several non EU countries that I had not been to so going through them I made sure to include their capitals. Only one, Bucharest, took me out of my way. I had to go through Turkey and I had not been to Ankara before and I was happy to see it was on the way. The only exception was that although we drove through Albania we were unable to include Tirana.

We decided on a sort of circular route starting with Dublin and then going via the west of France to Lisbon, Madrid and onwards in a partially anti clockwise way. Afterwards, although it made sense to go in a circle, I realized I had no idea how I chose anti-clockwise rather than the opposite. I think it was an effort to avoid the hottest part of Europe at the worst times and to make most use of daylight. Anyway it clearly did not meet these objectives.

The journey came out as having two different parts. The first involved mainly long drives with several days between seeing

13

doctors. For example it took a week between seeing the doctor in Dublin and the next one in Lisbon; and three days between Madrid and Rome. However, the second part, after Ljubljana was different and all journeys between EU capitals except Copenhagen and Amsterdam were one day and sometimes only a few hours; for example, the drive between Bratislava and Vienna was about two hours. I tried to make the drive like a holiday taking in interesting or pleasant places on the way such as Barcelona and Istanbul. Sometimes this idea was not successful in that our hotel in Barcelona was in an outer suburb on our route and we could not face driving into town that night or the cost of a return taxi. Other stays were better, such as Istanbul where we purposely had arranged two nights, but even when we stayed for only one night for example, in Ankara or Bucharest, the few hours we had were fascinating.

Driving in the south of Europe was complicated by having had to cross the Adriatic Sea and drive through or visit several islands including Sicily, Malta and Cyprus. It was necessary therefore to find out and book all these ferries. I discovered the details mainly on the Internet but had to use the phone a lot as some booking schedules were out of date or the lines were not working. I booked the ferry from Sicily to Malta on line and had to complete an enormous form. Passport numbers were no problem but I was a bit stuck when they asked for the car's chassis number, as I thought about thirty years ago cars stopped having a chassis (do they still have tappets and big ends?) and therefore presumably the number. I found some sort of number on the receipt and tried that but got a call saying that it was too short. Eventually I found a very long number on the windscreen and that seemed to satisfy the receptionist. For the form booking the Greek Island to the Turkish one there was a request for a photocopy of both sides of the credit card I used to pay and a copy of our identity cards. I knew of course I could have sent copies of our passports but I preferred to say proudly that we do not have identity cards in the UK and I still got my tickets. Sadly, as I learnt later in the south of Europe, it is not wise to take a light hearted approach to documentation. Mostly the receptionists in South Europe and Turkey spoke English and they answered the phone themselves without automatic switchboards. Imagine the pleasure of phoning an office and immediately talking to a human, who in many cases was the right person to deal with.

There were other problems however in the south. The ferry from Brindisi in the heel of Italy across the Adriatic could be booked only by fax and confirmed by deposit of money sent from my bank to theirs. My usual bank charges £35 for this but fortunately my savings bank, Smile, did it for about £13. I booked the ferry across the Aegean to the Greek island of Chios online three months in advance. I was told it would be confirmed but I heard nothing. Eventually I found the phone number on the website and after several calls, half of which terminated in the mantra that the computer was down, an email confirmation came.

There is only one ferry from Turkey to Cyprus that takes cars – indeed it seems to be the only one in Europe – and this holds for the 'right' Cyprus as well as the 'wrong' one. On the outward journey it leaves at midnight and takes from four to six hours depending who you ask. I booked the Turkish end and was told that I could not make a return booking but I must ring the Cyprus port to book that. The man was friendly but as we were about to finish I realized he had not asked for our names or the make of car, least of all the chassis number. When I chided him on this he assured me it was all correct and he had put it in a book. On phoning the Cyprus end it was similar but our names were taken. Fortunately Wendy teaches English as a foreign language to adults (EFL) and has charming Turkish governors in her class. They made enquires and discovered that this was the normal procedure and the ferries do not get fully booked.

Planning – Other problems

There were a couple of insurance type problems. Jaguar drivers, instead of being covered by the AA or RAC, are well looked after by Jaguar Assistance. However this does not cover all the countries in Eastern Europe. The only way round this was either to join the RAC or arrange cover for the whole of the trip with the RAC.

Both options were expensive and in the end I opted for the latter.

Jaguar themselves were helpful. When I told them what I was doing and asked for support they took the car into their factory for a week for a wash and brush up and four new tyres. A driver came down from Coventry took my car and left me a similar one.

More worrying was the car insurance. My car is insured through a broker with the Norwich Union and they do not cover Albania or Serbia. What to do? Phoning the Norwich Union was a load of laughs. I am sure this phrase is appropriate as their slogan is "make me happy". I used the number on my policy but after the usual option nonsense, combined with that dreadful warning that we may be recorded, I was told that this was Norwich Union Direct and my insurance was with the Norwich Union, a different company. I was transferred to them but they speak only to agents not to customers. I tried to say I wanted to speak to the top man, being Jewish I have been brought up with this ploy, but under no circumstances would the lady agree to listen to me. Instead she put me back to Norwich Union Direct and the man, after we agreed I was not insured with them, agreed to advise me, while, you understand, making it clear that really it was more than his job was worth. He told me Norwich Union, direct or otherwise, would not insure me for Albania and Serbia and that was it. He would not put me through to his supervisor let alone the top man because he knew what he would say. However my broker then worked on it and she found another company who were prepared to take me on, albeit with some swingeing excesses. Also they included a condition that the maximum number of days I could travel abroad was ninety nine, so after this holiday I would hardly be able to drive to France even, for nearly a year. I must say that I was disappointed at the attitude of the Norwich Unions. Obviously they were not going to change their policy just for me, but I had hoped they would understand the problem and put me in touch with colleagues who did operate in these two countries and help out a long-standing client.

There were a few other minor formalities such as getting International Driving Permits and EU health cards but these were no problem.

16

The Technical Side

Victoria, my younger daughter, works in medical market research and has had a lot of experience interviewing doctors and later in running projects. She advised me not to rely on taking notes which would be disruptive but to record the meetings. Modern equipment has changed a lot since tape recorders were used when I went to focus groups about thirty years ago. I bought a Sony recorder for just over £100. It is small and effective and very easy to use. The recordings download onto my computer in a trice and are clear to listen to. There were no problems in emailing the files home while I was away.

We did a role-play to test the equipment and the interview schedule with Victoria playing the doctor. Although somewhat artificial we showed the recording device was effective and easy to use and Victoria was able to give me constructive criticisms of my technique. The trial lasted a little over an hour. Although when meeting the doctors I recorded, with their consent, each interview except for one where the doctor thought, mistakenly, that her English was not good enough, I have not needed to transcribe these but keep them for reference.

When I returned to my hotel room immediately after each interview I dictated all that I had learned on to the machine and emailed it to Lucy, my other daughter, who typed it up and sent it back to me, usually within a day. When she was on holiday I employed a secretary. I then corrected the copy and emailed it to the doctor to make sure I had picked up the right facts. Often it took some time and pressure to get these returned but they came back with many helpful comments. Not every doctor replied. One did not use email so we discussed it by fax and phone and another used neither email nor fax and I sent his report by post but he did not reply.

Next, I realized I would need a laptop computer although apart from this project I have no use for one, as I am satisfied with my home desktop. Fortunately one of my sons-in-law has recently started a successful small business and forecast that he would need one in the autumn, so we paid half each. This enabled me to store my notes and photographs. It also gave me connection with the internet both to get information about countries, routes and even if there were any operas locally but also to send emails home to the family and friends. I had an arrangement with *GP* magazine, a weekly journal written, as the name implies, for general practitioners, to send them a series of five hundred word articles and photographs reporting my findings, the idea being that they would publish them as I went along. In fact the publication did not start until my return but I was very grateful to them and their associate editor, Jacki Buist who was extremely supportive, for agreeing to publish them.

The ability to access the Internet from the laptop was variable depending on the hotel. Ideally there was a free connection in the bedroom using either wifi or a cable connection. Sometimes there would be a charge. Although not desperately expensive the charge was always annoying and would sometimes be on a daily basis rather than a twenty four hour one. Where there was a charge it was often very difficult to set up. Sometimes instead of paying online I had to buy a scratch card with a numerical password which had to be revealed. If I scratched too hard, by the time all the gubbins was scraped off, some of the digits had gone as well and I had to start again thankfully at no extra charge. Sometimes the figures were so small it was hard to make them out. On these occasions, the hotels never accepted responsibility, saying they had contracted the service to an external organization. There was no pattern as to whether hotels would provide free internet connection. I stayed in a small hotel in an obscure town in Turkey with very little going for it but there was free internet in the bedroom, while in my luxury hotel in Amsterdam when, as it was towards the end we were splashing out, I was disappointed to be charged.

Another variation was where the internet location was located. In the expensive hotel we used in Rome it was free, but not available in the bedroom, and I had to use it in the lobby. There were occasions where an internet connection was provided but the staff could not get it to work. This happened in Turkey and Sweden. In Tasacu in Turkey the manager had a spare office with an internet connection and he allowed me to work there and connect up by laptop. I was very grateful to him.

Wendy wanted to make long phone calls to the family so we installed Skype which should have allowed her to make her calls cheaply through the computer. Unfortunately we usually had difficulty getting a satisfactory connection and we never really determined whether the equipment was faulty or we were not using it correctly. In the end we gave it up and wasted hundreds of pounds on our mobile phones.

The Holiday Side

The arranging of the meetings with the doctors, thinking about the structure of the interviews and the equipment, coupled with the journey with its insurance problems and booking the ferries made us so busy that we nearly forgot we were going on holiday for three months and it really was a holiday.

In towns where I had an interview we planned to stay two nights, usually three if one of them was a Sunday. This gave us some chance to see something at least of the town. It was frustrating when we stayed only one night when we were passing through cities such as Vienna, Barcelona or Belgrade.

Motoring holidays are a great pleasure to us and we often go to St Tropez for our summer holiday. If we are there for two weeks we will be away for three and drive both ways. I have found over the years that we have become unusual in this respect. Most of our friends going to the south of France, Spain or Italy prefer to fly-drive and say motoring to their destination is a complete waste of holiday time. Let us look at this waste of time. After work on the day before our holiday we drive to Dover and take a P&O ferry and have dinner in their Langan's Brassiere aboard. We then drive for five minutes to a comfortable Calais hotel. The next day, as we are already across the channel we have a good start. We will then drive to a town that sounds interesting, Nancy for example, and get there for lunch with plenty of time for a good look round in the afternoon. We make sure we have a good dinner, usually chosen from the Michelin Guide. Next day we finish the drive arriving in St Tropez in the mid afternoon. We then have our fortnight's holiday and decide where we would like to go to next. During this fortnight we drive around the area in our own car. Now I assume most people take care and trouble when they buy their car and want it as comfortable and as right for their needs as possible for the amount of money they are willing to spend. Associated with this for many is a sort of affection, if not love, for their car. What is the point of giving all this up for a strange hired one? I know that some holiday makers have never taken their car abroad and are frightened that driving a right-handed drive car on the right might appear to be a problem but I can assure them if they give it a go, within five minutes they will feel perfectly comfortable. If you want to take children and have more than three you will already own a vehicle with enough legal spaces for them and it is fantasy that, unless you child is unlucky enough to be car sick, children cannot enjoy long car journeys. When our children were small, although we played some games, they were entertained by audio tapes, *Joseph* and *Bang on a Drum* being favourites, and we all enjoyed singing along with them. Nowadays, they can have DVDs in the back and, if they want, their own individual ones. Lucy has four children and if she tries to hire a car not only does it have to be big enough but she has difficulty in arranging the provision of child safety seats for them all. Sometimes however they compromise and she or her husband Jeff will drive with two of the children and the other will take the others on a low cost airline, still therefore having the benefit of their own car.

The return drive could perhaps take us home after staying for a couple of days by a Swiss lake and then a couple of days in Chartres to explore the cathedral, every night making sure we are careful to choose our dinner. There are many variations for this third week and sometimes we go to the open-air opera in Verona.

Because we planned to stay in more than forty hotels I arranged with an agent from Wexas to do the booking and gave her a list of criteria. These started with the need for secure garaging for my car, facilities for the laptop and air conditioning. After fulfilling these, we

21

said we wanted each hotel to be as near to the centre of town as possible and not too expensive. I know that she found this to be an enormous task and was mostly successful, although probably tired near the end as in the later part of the journey fewer criteria were fulfilled.

After all these considerations how were we going to enjoy ourselves? We love frequent holidays together, but three months? At home we both had our careers which often required preparation, but for relaxation Wendy watches television, while I prefer to read. On holiday the high point of the day, as you must have discovered by now, is the evening meal which I find even more enjoyable if taken with lots of alcohol before, during and after and eaten as late as possible. We knew we could not keep this lifestyle going for so long and stay healthy.

I made some resolutions, including to avoid alcohol during the day, except the odd Guinness in Ireland, and I was mostly successful with this. We said we would try and eat earlier and healthier, although when it came to it we ate the same as we usually did on holiday. I intended to do thirty minutes exercise in the hotel gyms when available except on long driving days. This I am afraid never happened. We learnt to play backgammon and one of our friends, Val, who does tapestry as one of her many hobbies, bought a kit for Wendy and she spent time doing this. We both enjoy Su Doku. While I was with the doctors, Wendy usually arranged a sight-seeing trip of the town. Apart from the interviews, the journey was much like the sort of motoring holiday that we love.

Packing

We are not known for travelling light and usually the car is too full when we go to Europe for three weeks. This twelve week tour was obviously going to be a problem therefore, especially as I had to take my work bag, including my computer and the leads and other giblets that go with it. Wendy explained I did not need a clean shirt for every day and a further one for the evenings. And one hundred and sixty eight would take a lot of space, especially when combined with innumerable pairs of trousers, pants and socks. She said that we could wash the smalls on days where we were staying at least two nights and have the hotels launder the other clothes. I have no idea why we had not thought of this before but as a result we had fewer clothes than usual. We took a large and small case each and arranged our packing so that we needed only the small cases for our one night stops. We also had the computer case and a shared bag for books and shoes. All these fitted perfectly and symmetrically in the Jaguar boot and that was the end of the problem.

It is now time to look at the journey. The easiest way to do this is in the form of a travelogue describing our experiences of each country in turn. This is not a conventional description of the countries in that that sort of thing is available in all the guides and also there is no need to repeat well known-facts such as in Italy pasta is popular or in that in Scandinavia alcohol is expensive. No, I will confine myself to new impressions which may not have been noticed before, combined with thoughts about the pleasures and pains of travel and how to be prepared.

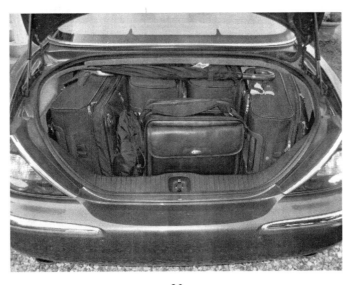

England and Wales

We left home on Saturday 17 June and made for Chester. This is an old Roman city with a surrounding wall and it is possible to walk on most of this seeing the city. At one point you can look down on to the main shopping street and the vision was rather like looking at a Lowry.

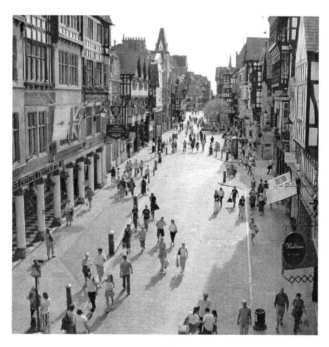

We decided to stay in a pub because not only, like bed and breakfasts, are they better value than hotels, they also cook a proper breakfast. I have never understood the paradox between the breakfasts in the expensive hotels and those in cheap pubs and B&Bs. In the former the cooked part is in a buffet, full of grease and going stale as you watch it. Many hotels cannot even provide a chef to cook the eggs freshly and to one's choice, merely providing a pot where removal of the lid reveals a load of greasy fried eggs dying on their feet, or what passes for feet in fried eggs. Contrast this to pubs and B&Bs where the waitress, who is often a very motherly landlady discusses what you want and then cooks it freshly for you at a fraction of the price.

It is because of this that we tend to avoid hotels in the UK and I would like to understand why people, except those on expense accounts, don't demand a freshly cooked breakfast for their money.

We looked up *The Good Pub Guide 2006* surely one of the most useful publications ever produced for travellers and day trippers in the UK, and found The Albion Pub. This was in an unpretentious building in a grotty street but otherwise provided all we could wish for. Let me explain by giving an example of how we were treated here, showing how these recommended pubs are worth their weight in gold. We had worried about how we were going to leave our loaded car safely overnight as there was no garage available. By a piece of good luck the parents, who we had never met, of our son Jeremy's best man Richard, lived just outside Chester. Jeremy asked Richard to ask his parents if we could leave our car at their house overnight. They not only agreed to this but Richard's father let me put my car in his locked garage and then he and his wife took us out for a splendid dinner just outside the town and then drove us back to the pub for the night. Anyway, the point of all this is that when we asked our landlady the next morning, after a good breakfast, to send for a taxi she insisted on taking us herself to Richard's parents' house where we were reunited with the Jaguar.

We then drove to Holyhead and had a pleasant voyage in a catamaran to Dublin. The drive from Chester was our only sojourn in Wales. I enjoyed this drive but I had to make an effort to stop my habitual worrying about who was paying for the road signs in Welsh as well as English. I have to dismiss such thoughts as, "Are there more non-English speaking Poles than Welsh in the province and therefore should we see trilingual signs?"

Ireland

We stayed in the Royal Hotel in O'Connell Street and this had all we wanted. It was right in the centre of town and had its own garage, although I had to pay to use the internet in our rather small bedroom. It was not expensive.

We had breakfast there and, although it was a buffet, it was redeemed by an egg wallah, a man of about fifty five who looked, from my experience of treating many Irish men, typically Irish and I realize this is a strange statement as I am not sure what that means, but anyway that was the warm feeling he gave me. He was slightly above middle height with greying hair, a rather wizened face and a kind smile. I must say he made lovely eggs.

The breakfast would have been good enough but disaster occurred. There was no Worcester sauce. I understand this liquid may be an acquired taste but I can hardly ever remember having a greasy fried breakfast without it, even as a child at home, and I was bereft. There was brown sauce and ketchup but these were totally useless. I was surprised that they could not find some as, even if their guests make up an eccentric clientele who have breakfast without it, there must be some available in the bar for the tomato cocktail. I must say the staff looked high and low but no luck. However the chef promised it for the morrow and the pride with which he proffered it then was a joy to behold.

As far as I can observe, few people are fussy about this sort of thing but it is important to me. It must come from my upbringing in which at home, apart from the sauce mentioned, we always had mint sauce with roast lamb and mustard with roast beef and steak. I love pink roast lamb but the complete taste for me is a blend of the meat and mint and one is lost without the other.

The mustard is a tricky area. In my childhood the only mustard we had was Colman's English Mustard which in those days was only the powdered variety, which is made up with the addition of a little water. While I was growing up Colman's changed the name to Superfine Mustard and marketed Colman's English Mustard as some ready-made concoction in a jar. I will not say a word against it except that it is quite different and I do not like it. Nor incidentally do I like any other.

I have got round the problem by always carrying my own mustard powder with me. I used to keep it in the original tin in the car and if I ordered beef I would ask the waiter to make it up for me explaining the recipe. Once in Monterey in California this went wrong and the waitress brought a large glass of pale yellow liquid with a cocktail cherry on top. "Gee," she said, "I love the English accent," but I think she meant more than that.

I then changed my technique. I dispense portions of the powder into plastic 35 mm film box containers and to prevent accidents wrap each one in a polythene bag so kindly given by banks to store coins. I then take the lid off and pour in a small amount of water, shake vigorously and Bob's your uncle – I love that expression – there is the perfect mustard. Occasionally containers get left behind and in the age of digital photography I am aware that they may stop being made, so I replenish them from time to time. About two years ago, while having dinner in a Bulgarian coastal resort on a Black Sea cruise we found a souvenir shop which processed photographs open until late in the night. The shop keeper and we shared no common language but I was able to explain what I wanted although not unfortunately the reason for the need. It always seems rather difficult to account for my wish to walk around a Bulgarian Black Sea resort late in the evening begging used film containers.

My brother-in-law had a similar although not identical problem and it took me some years to persuade him to solve it. He is very fond of a drink called lager-and-lime and is always disappointed if the restaurant, pub or whatever has the former without the latter. He now has the solution with him, both metaphorically and literally.

I first went to Dublin as a medical student in the fifties to do my maternity training. It had a reputation as a centre of excellence but this was merely due to the fact that because of the very high birth rate they delivered a lot of babies. However, I regret that far from being excellent their methods were cruel and barbaric. Obviously that was many years ago and I hope that the Rotunda now is as good as the best. I enjoyed the four weeks I had stayed there living in the hospital and it was good to see it again.

The day after arriving in Dublin I drove for my appointment to a suburb called Naas. I thought I had allowed plenty of time but Dublin is booming and I was held up by road works. The surgery was in a new development unknown to Gladys and I had difficulty finding it. I was late and terrified I would miss the appointment. However Dr Shearer was very nice about it and the interview was most successful. At the end of the meeting he invited Wendy and me out to dinner in the evening. He suggested a fish restaurant, 'The Mackerel,' in the centre of Dublin near our hotel and the fish soup was better than in the south of France, as was the seafood platter. This restaurant is in the upstairs of Bewley's Coffee Shop, a traditional haunt that was part of a chain going back to 1840. Sadly, this restaurant is now closed. I hope it is not pseud because the coffee house part downstairs gives the impression that this is how gentlemen would have done business and discussed politics a hundred years ago. As did most other doctors who took us out, they hosted the evening. This was something I had not expected in advance and it helps to make me long to see the European doctors come to London where I can not only meet them again but return some hospitality. Spending the evening with Ann and Dermot made a lovely end to our first city stay.

Incidentally while I was with Dermot for my interview, Wendy went on a walking tour of Dublin and this set the pattern for her during many of my visits. She nearly always returned enthusiastic.

Portugal

It took a week before I saw my next doctor as we had to drive to the south-west of Ireland, and then take a ferry to Brittany in north-west France. The voyage was unpleasant partly because the sea was rough overnight and also because the cabin in the Irish Ferry from Rosslare to Cherbourg was surprisingly small and ill-equipped. It was difficult for us to stand in a two berthed cabin where there were bunk beds but virtually no floor space so we paid extra for a four berth cabin where we could not exactly spread ourselves but there was a little more space. The shower room was horrible, very small with a tiny towel and liquid soap hidden away in the shower. The toilet tissue was a pile of small sheets of paper about the size of NHS prescriptions. With the fares they charge they would normally be expected to provide better, but they must still suspect the passengers of stealing everything not screwed down. In the evening in the lounge we watched part of the World Cup football, when England drew two all with Sweden. We could see only bits because the signal kept going but we knew we would be in the finals.

Things looked up when we reached Plancoët in Brittany, where we stayed in a hotel which has to be anyone's favourite hotel, although strictly speaking I believe it is a one rosette restaurant with rooms. The food and service are something to look forward to. We had been there before in 1998. If you order lobster they put pelican type bibs round you, one of the many thoughtful gestures. The bedrooms are large, beautiful and every convenience is thought of as though you were staying in Chewton Glen or *Le Manoir a' Quatre Saisons* but at a significantly more affordable price.

We then drove through France and Spain to Lisbon. This was a mixture of easy motorway driving by day and good food in the evenings. We had a two day break in Salamanca as it was on the way and Victoria had been there to University. It is a beautiful town with a spectacular Plaza Major together with the University and the cathedral. We were taken out by a family of Victoria's friends whom we had met in the past and they showed us much of the university that we would not find on our own. In Salamanca we stayed in a Parador and as we expected our bedroom was bigger than our lounge at home.

It was easy driving in Portugal and the roads were dual carriageway if not motorway where sometimes they charge and sometimes not. Occasionally they are not sure, when you come to a toll station at the start of a section where you collect a ticket and then nothing more happens, neither the ticket is asked for nor a toll paid.

In the restaurants we were given a big 'feel good' factor. We had an omelette and chips for lunch near our hotel. It was the day of the round before the quarter finals (eighth finals?) of the World Cup. In the afternoon I walked up to one of the big posh hotels – I think it was the Sheraton but it could have been the Meridian – and sat in the bar where they were showing England playing Ecuador with a Portuguese commentary and I was relieved we won, with Beckham scoring the only goal.

In the evening we had dinner nearby in a restaurant overlooking the Eduard VII Park. As at lunch time, the waiters really wanted us to feel at home. I thought I would try the "When in Rome…" routine and had a white Port as an aperitif. It was sweeter than I remembered but worth a try. After an excellent dinner I had some red port and long after the bill came the waiters kept refilling my glass. During dinner Portugal were playing Holland and fortunately they won by scoring only one goal. The walk back from the restaurant to the hotel must have been like London on VE night except for the cars. Everyone was screaming with joy and the cars, all festooned with Portuguese flags, were hooting non-stop. The happiness was infectious and we were glad for them that they won, although this as you probably know was not an emotion that persisted beyond the end of the week. What I liked about this feeling of joy was that you felt glad to be part of it, and there was no feeling of menace that you can sometimes feel after a similar event in England.

We stayed in a small Best Western Hotel, also near the park. I remember it had a small but perfectly reliable lift. Lifts in hotels are funny places, apart from their electronic idiosyncrasies. Ours were all automatic and came with little delay. There were no problems, but what is the etiquette if you are not alone? Especially if one other person joins you? Are you supposed to pretend he is not there and look the other way or should you discuss the weather? My late mother-in-law would talk to everyone and I used to tease her that by the time they reached the ground floor she would know how often a fellow passenger made love and in which position. It still amuses me that when a lift is on the way down if it stops, say, at the third floor a fellow passenger will bound out thinking he has reached ground level, only to be hauled back by his wife.

The next morning I walked from the hotel to see Dr Mendes who is president of the Portuguese college of GPs, in the college office. It was an honour to meet someone so distinguished and after a detailed interview he sent me with an assistant by taxi to meet GPs in their enormous health centre.

Later in the day we went to see the sights we remembered from past visits, including the public elevator designed in 1902 by Gustave Eiffel of Parisian Eiffel Tower fame and had dinner near the harbour.

Spain

Although we went to Madrid to see my Spanish doctor after we had been to Lisbon we had of course to drive through Spain first from France. We therefore had two Spanish phases, pre Portuguese and post Portuguese. We had been rather ambitious on the day we left France for Spain because we went from Brittany to Bilbao: a journey of a little over five hundred miles. It was of course all motorways and not nearly as hard a day as it appears. Bilbao is well served by motorways but leaving the city my petrol warning light was on and while negotiating the knot of highways and slip roads I could find no filling stations. The range given on the car computer was down to zero and the needle firmly stuck in the red on the petrol gauge, rather like Mr. Micawber's bank account. I did not say anything to Wendy and in the Jaguar the passenger can see neither the petrol level nor the warning light. As you can imagine, I was working up a great sweat, as I knew the car may stop at any moment and I had no idea of the process or time it would take to get rescued. I also was aware that we had five hundred miles to go to reach our booked hotel and stay on schedule. The sight of the garage at last gave me such a feeling of joy. I assume it must be similar to what a tennis player feels on winning the Wimbledon finals.

As a result of this episode we resolved for the rest of the trip to keep the tank more than a third full. There was no one country where fuel stations were hard to come by but you never could tell. Often there would be long stretches of road, especially off motorway, when we seemed to go more miles without seeing one than the car's supply with the warning light on could cope with.

I felt guilty that we got into this position because something similar had happened to us while driving in the Dordogne area in France the previous year. We were in a town on a Sunday when the fuel warning light came on. When this happens Gladys is helpful as she displays all the local petrol stations on the map on her screen. (I am puzzled as to why I did not use this facility in Bilbao – it may be that I was furiously concentrating on finding the right lanes in their motorway system.) We thought that should solve the problem but as we approached each one we found it closed, and this included the supermarkets. Literally we did not know what to do. We came by a smart hotel and after a brief conversation we half-kidnapped the concierge's assistant, a boy of about seventeen. He took us to a supermarket which, as is common in France, had Sunday closing. He showed me the places to operate the pump with my credit card. I tried this but it would not work. In the end we all waited, Wendy, the young assistant and I, until a car came to fill up. Together we were able to explain to the driver the problem and I gave him twenty euros in cash so he could put this money's worth of fuel into my car and add the cost to his credit card bill. Fortunately that was enough to get me to a service station on a motorway, firstly, of course, having returned a well-tipped youth back to his hotel.

The beauties of Spain are well known but to me a special feature is the times of their meals. I know they do not suit everyone but to me they are really civilized. It is nice to know that you can sit down to lunch at four o'clock but more important is that dinner is at about nine 'clock or even later. This makes for a long day finishing up with a rest and then dinner with no sense of rush.

Wendy and I tend to eat late but unfortunately I am told as one gets older the digestion will not stand up to going to bed soon after a meal. Although we have not noticed this, many of our equally aging friends have so, if we want company we have to be flexible and eat earlier.

Being persuaded by friends is not the same as being forced by restaurants. In Phoenix, Arizona once we were lucky to be served at half past eight and even then we could not get the rib we hoped for and were the last diners there.

When going to the theatre we prefer dinner afterwards as, if the play is good, you need time to discuss it, and if bad or boring at least you have something to look forward to. There is no problem about this in London nor of course Spain but recently I went to Aberdeen for the opera for two nights and it was almost impossible to get a meal afterwards; certainly, the Scottish locals had never heard of such a thing. Fortunately the local Indian, willingly, and Chinese reluctantly, were able to help out.

Madrid must be booming because everywhere you look there were cranes and the whole city seemed to be one vast building site. Some of the new architecture strikes you as you approach. Just near our hotel a little out of the city centre was an edifice rather like two giant dominoes; one on either side of the road leaning towards each other.

Gladys however, let us down here because she took us to an unfinished structure outside the city. This was done by programming in the address. I tried again with the postcode but, as in other countries, unique postcodes cover a larger area then in England and we still had difficulty in finding the hotel when we reached the right area.

I saw a GP called Dr Engels and he seemed bilingual. His daughter was attending Glasgow University. He was kind enough to pick me up from my hotel at four o' clock and take me to his modern health centre some way out of town. In the morning Wendy and I had taken a taxi to the centre of Madrid and seen the Royal Palace, had coffee in the Plaza Major and lunch in the Plaza Colone, where Victoria had worked for a year. I had noticed both when in Dublin and Madrid the mornings before interviews were rather spoilt by an increasing feeling of nervousness. It was not that I was frightened of the doctors, just that something would go wrong with the meeting. As time progressed these feelings never really went away.

Italy

From Madrid, which we had found a nightmare to drive round, and after an easy journey to the suburbs of Barcelona, we went to the south of France where we sunbathed on the beach at La Napoule for a few hours on the way to Rome.

As you drive into Northern Italy the first thing you notice are the motorways. Because of the mountains they are magnificent feats of engineering with bends and tunnels and as Italy is a rich country there is a large volume of traffic, creating a mismatch, and there were many traffic jams. As in parts of France they have this curious habit of having paying sections for just a few kilometres, so the passenger who, in an English car is the one who has to deal with the toll booths (and of course is also the co driver), has to keep waking up to pay. At least they now take credit cards. I remember in about 1984 driving from the French Riviera into Italy and having a long hold up in a tunnel. When we finally reached the front we found it was due to a toll station, which took no credit cards, and we had to pay something like 8,657 lire and wait for our change to be counted. South of Rome the motorways are quiet but are mostly being rebuilt, so the roadworks were in long stretches.

Some tolls were automatic and tickets were taken at two levels, the higher for lorry drivers. At one point in Sicily, where people seem shorter, the lower level slot was not working so drivers had to get out of their cars and reach up. Some poor Sicilian could not make it and, being tall, I was pleased to be able to do something useful and assist him.

The signposts on the motorways are not nearly as good as the UK or France and on ordinary roads they are useless. As you come to a fork in the road there will be a list of towns, each with its own board facing one way and another facing the other. There is no time to read them as you drive past so you have to slow down and, if the list is long, stop, incurring the wrath of the drivers behind. I have always noticed this system in Italy but what has surprised me is that the Italians haven't, and in spite of international travel there are no indications of any pending improvement.

Perhaps this is a good place to pause and think about another road sign problem everywhere, including even the UK and France, both countries in my opinion having the clearest. This is the putting-of-one-sign-in-front-of-another syndrome. I am sure you know what I mean. The sign you are looking for saying "Slopton-on-the-Push turn right" is obscured by another sign about no loading in Lent. What fool put that up? There must be jobsworths in each council throughout Europe responsible for road signs and only one needs to notice the problem and publish it in his trade magazine and they may all get the point. As well as signs blocking signs there is the problem of foliage in the way, and often in season you cannot find your way because of a large branch obscuring the important bit. I suggest each council, prefecture or what-you-will recruits a person normally selling *The Big Issue*, or local equivalent, equips him with a pair of strong shears and a portable ladder and tells him to cycle around the whole borough and cut off without mercy anything in the way. This job should include the right to lop off any branches or foliage protruding from private properties, although perhaps it would be polite to give some warning first.

Although Rome is a big city to drive through it is not as difficult as Madrid. The centre was quieter than expected. I wanted to reach our hotel in time for the quarter final of the World Cup, which was on I think at four o'clock in the afternoon. It was quite a drive from Menton and it meant missing lunch but we arrived at the hotel with five minutes to spare. Wendy checked in, a porter took the luggage, a valet parker took away the car and the concierge directed me to an American bar nearby where they were showing the match in English. I just made it and was served some beer as I slowly felt my heart sinking, watching Rooney sent off and England being knocked out by Portugal, about whom we had such warm feelings, and by penalties at that. That, I must admit, was the end of the World Cup for me.

Our hotel was pleasant enough but being in the centre it was expensive. Our friends Sylvia and Edgar joined us in Rome and we had a lot of fun, especially with the meals. In Rome I had arranged to see a lady doctor, Luisa Valle, who had invited us to stay with her but as this was one of the occasions when a couple of our friends had decided to join us for the weekend we declined. To compensate for this she and her husband, Claudio, took us, together with Sylvia and Edgar, to a restaurant where they were obviously known. The meal was fabulous. You know that in an Italian restaurant for the first course you have a choice of antipasta or a starter portion of pasta. Well here it did not work like that. The meal started with a variety of antipasti which is the Italian way of saying Mixed hors d'oeuvres. Then followed a generous portion of pasta

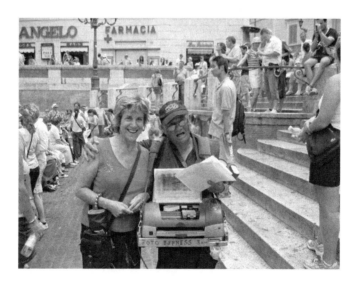

before we got down to the serious business of the main course of lamb. This was followed by various desserts including fruit and ice-cream. Fortunately, although we seemed to have eaten an enormous meal we did not feel unpleasantly bloated afterwards. But oh! so happy.

We had been to Rome before and had seen many of the sights but when we returned to the Trevi fountain we were interested to see a photographer. As well as having a digital camera he had a printer suspended from his neck like an ice-cream tray on a theatre usherette. He was able to take punters' pictures and print them out immediately and this was accompanied by the warmest smile you can imagine, he just had that sort of face. The picture was fine and takes pride of place in Wendy's scrap book.

All this was on a Sunday. The next morning Wendy, Sylvia and Edgar went sight-seeing while I drove to a suburb of Rome, where I met Luisa in the local hospital car park from where she drove me to her surgery.

Malta

The next doctor to see was in Malta. To drive there we had to go through Sicily first, crossing the Straits of Messina in a short but picturesque ferry journey. After an overnight stay in Sicily we drove to the south of the island for the ferry to Malta. I regret the experience was not good; although the boat was comfortable the formalities were almost a nightmare (the real nightmare came later with the Turkish borders). However there was no excuse because Italy and Malta are in the EU, just the same as Britain and France.

The troubles started at the entrance to the part of the harbour, where on each side of the gate was a sign saying "Entrance to ferry for Malta". Unfortunately, there was a clear No Entry sign on the gate. What to do? We were determined not to miss the ferry so we drove through and there were few people around to whom we could ask. We arrived at a T-junction with an office at the end. We were hoping to check in when we saw it was a snack kiosk. To turn right or left was I thought fifty-fifty but Wendy had seen a ship moored on the right as we drove in and on turning that way she was proved correct. We drove up to a beautiful ship with the car ramp open and waiting apparently for us. It did not work like that. First we had to queue to register. This took a few minutes although the receptionist told us someone had forgotten our tickets and had we paid? Never a good start. Anyway, she must have thought we looked honest and gave us three boarding cards, one for each of us, and one for the car. We were told that the driver takes the car on and the passenger walks on separately. We discussed where we would meet. Wendy disappeared into a passenger passport registration booth carrying of course not only her boarding card but the car's also. I sat in the car wondering whether to drive on when I noticed a brightly uniformed official going to each driver in turn. He was very pleasant to me and when he had finished I was about to start the engine when I thought I heard him say I must wait for the soldier and this proved to be the case. Soldiers with caps, drab uniforms and wielding rifles were going round the preceding cars making drivers open the boot. Fortunately when he came to me he was all smiles, glanced at my passport and waved me on and Hey Presto! I was aboard. Yet another official inspected the boarding card and was disconcerted to find I could not produce one for the car. Rather unkindly, I saw that as her problem in that there was no room to turn round and drive off again but anyway Wendy, seeing that she had the missing pass, walked quite illegally down to the car deck and saved the situation.

The boat left on time but spent twenty minutes mooring in Valletta and instead of, as on P&O ferries at Dover or Calais, being told to go back to our cars the whole ship's staff, who were mostly Polish and Romanian young ladies who did not speak English, formed a guard across the stairway down to the vehicle deck. It took ages before cars could drive off and as we were about to start another uniformed officer in a smart hat went round all the vehicles asking for passports and Green Cards. Green Cards are no longer used in the EU but, contrary to advice, I insisted on having one as we were going to non-EU states. Ours, as we thought it would not be needed, was packed in a suitcase but the man insisted on seeing it. When we found it I explained to him that it was neither interesting nor necessary but while agreeing he said to see it was his instruction and there was no way round that. I had of course realized by this time my car was the only British one on the boat, if not in the whole country. As I left the port there were several elderly men copying the car numbers on to scraps of paper the way they write down your voting number outside polling booths. I never discovered the reason for this. Perhaps Malta is still expecting an invasion from Italy? Finally in this episode as I drove out there were no "Drive on the left" signs visible and having been driving in Europe for over two weeks there was nearly a nasty accident. The return journey to Sicily was much the same, with no information that the car should be left on the main road and then we had to walk back along the gate to have our passports checked and obtain boarding passes and then go our separate ways again on to the ship.

The whole business was extremely unpleasant, made worse by the fact that it was unnecessary. You do not get all this nonsense when travelling by ferry between England and France and, like them, we do not have a Shengen agreement, in which frontier formalities are waived between EU countries. Although blame has to be apportioned, it is difficult to know where. The ferry company would say that the troubles were due to the Maltese and Italian governments and each government would blame the other and the company.

Wherever the fault lies, there are some conclusions to be drawn. The first is that the directors and managers of Viameux , the ferry owners, need to study the P&O operation between Dover and Calais and learn how it should be done.

The second person to blame is the Minister for Europe who either knows nothing about this or has not bothered to correct it. He could explain to the Maltese government that in the EU, Green Cards are not thought necessary and vehicle registration documents are rarely carried in the West at least. He should teach the Maltese authorities that to share the privileges of the EU they must make sure that travellers have an easy, understandable and safe experience with no more formalities than necessary for safety. Some of the troubles may be down to the Italian authorities but I am influenced by my experience of no trouble at their other EU borders. I cannot exonerate them entirely because when taking the ferry from Sicily to Albania, while thinking I would not make a fuss because this was not an EU frontier, I could not help wondering why all passengers had to queue standing in a hot unair-conditioned office for over half an hour, many carrying babies, to see a lone passport officer sitting behind a cubby hole in his air-conditioned room.

In Malta we had time only for Valletta, which is a pleasant town with lovely old buildings mixed with the squalid. There is a big café-cum-bar spread across both sides of the main street just before the square. One side was an air-conditioned pleasant room; the other was outside with plenty of sunshades. The place was filthy, the floor not having been swept, the waiter laconic and surly and the food poor. At St Juliens we went to a restaurant, which was better but not great and again not really friendly. The taxis do not have meters and taking it all in together it has to be faced that Malta is not ready for the tourist trade and if you are looking for a good holiday on a sunny Mediterranean Island it might be better to wait for a few years.

However, we stayed in the Meridian Phoenicia, a large hotel at the edge of the town centre. This is not where the holiday action is but the hotel is luxurious with large lounges and a big well-equipped bedroom. We have stayed here before and it was no let-down to return to it. For me, if I had to go to Malta again, this is where I would stay.

My doctor in Malta was Jean Carl Soler and he worked in Attard, a few kilometres from Valetta. Although he was partner in a private practice he knew all about the state system. He is an academic type and a member of WONCA. He was one of the first doctors to respond to my initial email sent through the RCGP.

There is a curious phenomenon in Valletta. The language as expected is Maltese, with many of the population speaking English as a second language. This is not surprising as it was a British colony until the seventies. However nearly all the signs in and around the town were in English, with absolutely no Maltese. This meant all the shop fronts, big or small, and signposts. In fact, the only Maltese on view was on the small and inadequate nameplates of roads. This seemed even more eccentric than places like Wales and Ireland where the road signs are in the language that almost everyone uses as well as, hopefully, their local one.

Greece

To get to Greece we went back from Malta to Sicily with the same hassles on the otherwise comfortable ferry, and then from the toe to the heel of Italy where we took another overnight ferry to Albania from Brindisi across the Adriatic. This was poor but tolerable. Cabins were similar to those on the Irish Ferries, although without asking we were upgraded to a four-berthed cabin, also very small. If possible, the bathroom was even smaller and although a shower was provided, as far as I could tell you would have to stand in the loo to use it. One small piece of sheeting was provided to take the place of towels. There was a self-service restaurant but the food is best left as indescribable.

Arriving in Albania by the car ferry, the frontier formalities at the port were formal but not tedious and organized in a logical way of passport and customs and it all took a few minutes. Albania was not as sinister as its past reputation might lead one to expect, although I have to admit to having dealt with few Albanians. I remember reading an AA guide book to Europe about thirty years ago and it warned that beards and bibles were forbidden. Things have almost certainly changed now but as we did not carry either we never found out. I assumed from *Cosi Fan Tutti* that the Albanian men would all have large moustaches but this turned out to be a misconception.

Anyway, after leaving the ferry we were soon on our way down the coast road. This was well made at first and passed inlets and over mountains, making great viewing. Unfortunately, after a few miles, the road stopped being made up and there were large potholes. There was room for only one car and many hairpin bends. There was always the risk of finding another car or lorry coming round the other way in the middle of the road. Sections had no crash barriers at the edges, even high up, and the driving became more frightening than enjoyable. What, according to the computer, should have taken two hours lasted six. We spoke to people at a garage in sign language and they were friendly, giving us a bottle of water and directing us on our way.

I suppose each country has its own curiosities and Albania's was the number of Mercedes cars. Although there was no question of traffic jams where we were, there was a steady stream of cars and my impression was that about ninety percent were Mercedes, evenly split amongst old, middle age and new. I guess that about eight percent more were Volkswagens and the remaining two percent a mixture. However, to make it more interesting, we saw quite a few donkeys on the road, some pulling carts.

The roads in Albania were clearly signposted. It was a pity we did not go to a town as it would have been an interesting experience but sadly and probably mistakenly we had arranged to get out of the country as soon as possible.

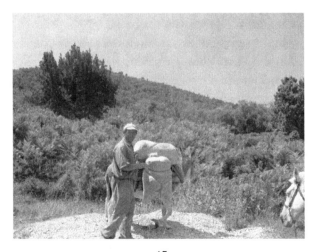

We crossed into Greece and found wide roads but apart from a spectacular new road bridge over the Gulf of Corinth not much else. We needed petrol and lunch and stopped at the first garage with credit card signs. After filling the tank, the owner told me his machine did not work and I must pay cash. He was not bothered that we hardly had any, he told me there was an ATM in a village three kilometres away and his daughter would drive me there. Wendy stayed to try to get some food for us and I went in this girl's old car to the bank which was actually fifteen kilometres away. She drove at one hundred and thirty kilometres an hour, the speed limit being one hundred, and as well as not wearing her seat belt she was talking to her hand held mobile phone. I supposed I should have been frightened but I could not help admiring her confidence and audacity. It all turned out well and at the end I paid the garage and had a fried egg sandwich which, as it was the only food I had had that day and it was now four o'clock, tasted delicious.

Athens, of course, is worth seeing because of the relics of the past. Our hotel was near the Acropolis and we could just see the Pantheon from on the top. We went to the swimming pool on the roof of a nearby hotel from where you could get quite a good, although distant, view. It was sad when lowering my eyes from the Acropolis I saw all the houses below and all I can say is that the architecture was shocking; it looked just like a shantytown and was the poorest place we had seen. I would like to know in which era it was built and what Athenians think of it.

We saw the changing of the guard outside the palace. It was very elaborate, almost like a ballet. Two soldiers turned towards or away from each other at appropriate times and then marched to meet using intricate steps with the right foot going high in the air while the left almost appeared to shuffle at the same time. Simultaneously one arm appeared to be doing the crawl. While admiring all this I had a wistful feeling that they were guarding a palace without a King or Queen and I felt so grateful that the UK is still romantic enough to keep its Royal Family.

The doctor I had arranged to meet I interviewed the next day. He is George Panagopoulos, a pediatrician. He had told me on the phone that there were very few GPs in Greece so he would find out all about primary care in the country in advance and so be well briefed to help me. When I told him I was surprised he was willing to take so much trouble he said he would enjoy doing it as he would like to learn more about the Greek system himself. In the event he had made copious and very useful notes clearly explaining a very complicated system. He said travel round Athens could be tricky and he came by train from his suburb to talk to me in my hotel where the management were kind enough to loan me an interview room without charge.

Any description of Greece would be a good place to mention my obsession about smoking which through clinical experience I share with many doctors. I am afraid the subject recurs as is the way with obsessions, and Greece is a good place to start because, as in Turkey, there is so much of it that even the busy streets smell of it.

I do not like the smell of cigarette smoke and prefer to eat in restaurants where I am protected from it. I sort of welcomed the law in England banning smoking in pubs and restaurants among other places, although it seems a pity that there should not be rooms in large enough establishments where smokers could indulge. Incidentally, I do not understand smokers; either they must be very thick to reject the overwhelming evidence of its dangers, or drug addicts, which implies they are sicker then they realize. They do not of course sense the unpleasant smell they exude to non-smokers and consequently how unattractive they are. For them to call doctors anti-smoking fascists demonstrate a frightening ignorance of what smoking does and what fascists did.

As will be remembered this journey was made in 2006, before the new smoking laws were introduced anywhere in the UK. It was pleasant to go into restaurants and bars in Ireland and Italy for example and know there was no need to worry who was sitting at the next table. In Spanish restaurants, few people smoked but there was often one which was enough to spoil the atmosphere for the surrounding tables.

Few if any countries ban smoking at tables out of doors and this is a mistake. Much as I do not want to persecute smokers, I should point out that the smoke from a nearby table out of doors wafts over the other tables in the same way as being inside.

As I said, I was pleased to be in non-smoking restaurants in Italy (inside) but the government was brave to bring in the law because so many people smoke. I saw a security guard, with a bank van, complete with dark glasses, revolver in his hand and cigarette in his mouth. On a ferry to Sicily in the bar, which was of course non-smoking, nobody did except the staff, including the chef and waiter. They were at it all the time, although to be fair it was quiet and there were no customers. When we docked, the matelot organizing ropes and doorways had a permanent cigarette in his mouth. If this project discovers nothing else it may find the cause of global warming. In Greece and Turkey and presumably many unvisited countries most of the men and many of the women, from before breakfast until late at night, hold small fires in their hands or mouths heating up the atmosphere.

I have no problem with smokers getting treatment on the NHS. Smokers are still humans and I can see no reason to discriminate against them unless the smoking makes the condition unlikely to be treatable. I know they often bring the illness on themselves but after all, they contribute much in tobacco tax and are less likely to draw their state pension for long.

Cyprus

I assume that the European Union admitted Cyprus as a practical joke, thinking that the hurdles that seemed to have been erected especially to screw up my plans would give them some amusement. Certainly if your humour is to see people slipping on banana skins, you would have had fun with this lot of problems.

Firstly, it is not even in Europe. Although Wikipedia says it is in Eurasia, wherever that is, a glance at the map would have shown them that it is off the coast of the Asian part of Turkey and is clearly therefore not in Europe.

Secondly it is not one country, but two. The part I wanted, which is the official EU country although in the wrong continent, takes up two thirds of the island; unfortunately for me, as we shall see, the wrong two thirds. We will call this the Cypriot part. What you call the other third depends on your point of view. The Cypriots from the Cypriot part call it the Turkish-occupied part. Turkey calls it an independent republic but the rest of the world disagrees and mumbles something vague and diplomatic in foreign. For simplicity, and I am implying no views in this, we will call it the Turkish part.

Anyway as the Cypriot Cypriots do not recognize the Turkish part, they have made a law that foreigners cannot enter their country from there. Unfortunately as I have said they have the wrong bit because, being in the South, the only way to get there with a car is from the north. There is no other way. Believe me, I have tried. Browsing the internet, I discovered car ferries going to the south

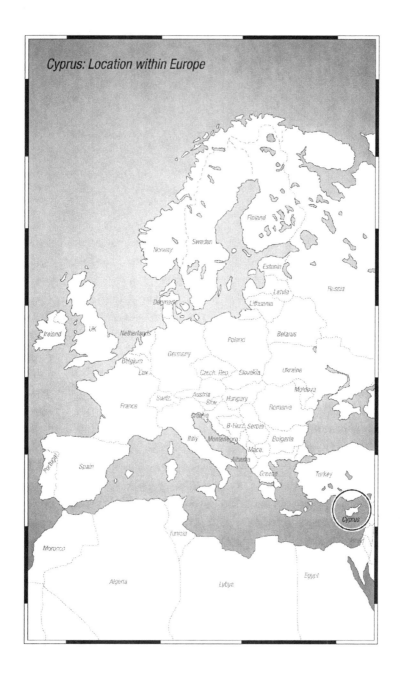

Cyprus: Location within Europe

from Israel and Greece but in fact they have not run for some years. The website for 'Salamis' lines gives the timetable for ferries from Greece to Cyprus for 2002. Freight ships would have been an option but prohibitively expensive.

I tramped round London calling at various touring offices including the Turkish and Cypriot ones who were not helpful, and the Turkish Cypriot ones who were. I spoke to doctors in Cyprus and wrote to the British foreign secretary who did not reply until I wrote to my MP, Andrew Dismore, who pushed things along, the Cypriot High Commission and the Minister of Health in Nicosia. It was the Ministry of Health who gave me permission to interview a doctor in Nicosia and without this I was told no GP would see me. As we have seen, I had a letter from her giving me the name and details of the doctor to contact.

What I learnt was that, although nobody claimed to know, most people's feelings were that the law remains but is variably enforced. Even if they would not let me drive through, I was prepared to garage my car in the northern side of Nicosia – the border runs thorough the capital – and then hope to walk through. There were plenty of problems before reaching this stage.

The extra time and distance caused by Cyprus being in the wrong place was considerable. My interview with George Panagopoulos in Athens had been on Tuesday 11th July. Next day we started our journey to Nicosia and took a ferry from Piraeus to Chios, just off the coast of Turkey. On Thursday 13th July we sailed to Turkey and were outside the EU until Monday 31st July when I arrived, now with Rod, in Slovenia, having seen only the doctor in Nicosia in the meantime. To be fair, I had factored a spare six days for Turkey, three of which we spent at a seaside resort before travelling to Cyprus and three in another afterwards. The reason for this, that there were so many things that could go wrong with our health, the car, bureaucrats and crooks that I felt the spare days would give me a chance to catch up if I got behind because many of the appointments had been hard to fix and had critical timing. In the event we were lucky and these spare days were not needed.

The worst problems were with the Turkish ferry and land

frontiers. The first ferry was from Chios to Cesme and this was not too bad. The other passengers were three groups of tourists, all in bright new cars. Although we were surprised as to how many offices we had to go through at the port we were accompanied by a smiling official who conduced us through.

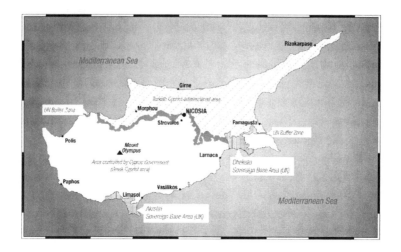

Cyprus

The next ferry was from Turkey at Tasacu to Girne in northern Cyprus. We thought this would be a breeze, especially as we were going from Turkey to the Turkish part. The process firstly involved going to several offices for passport control and customs. We had to show our passports about six times and each time they were studied in detail. There was frequent interest in the Vehicle Registration Document and we had to find and surrender a copy of a document we had been given on entry to Turkey at Cesme. Finally we started boarding the boat when a policewoman indicated we were missing a stamp on my passport, and said we had to go back. I refused to move the car but we walked back to the series of offices, trying to find where to go and, after several attempts, each time rather embarrassingly pushing to the front of the queue, we found the right place, got the passport stamped and returned to the car. This time the policewoman told us between puffs that something else was missing and we had to go back again. After the same procedure we were sent back a third time and then finally boarded this basic and smelly ferry. At no stage during all this did we find anyone who spoke English or French.

Inside there was one big non-smoking lounge. Although a change from cigarette smoke, the smells were of toasted cheese and meat sandwiches, the only food they had, which were revolting with a horrible taste, leaving a foul feeling in the mouth. It was warm outside and it was possible to share a bench with the smokers. The ferry was scheduled to leave at midnight but actually left at three o'clock which I gather is the norm.

Arriving in Northern Cyprus it was all the same but we by now were expecting problems and were more prepared. At one stage during the whole procedure we were sent to a plush air-conditioned office to meet a gentleman, wearing a suit and tie, who gave us a lovely smile and offered us coffee. We could not find out why we were asked to do this, as we seemed to be the only ones. One customs officer spoke English, which eased the process. We were now in Cyprus but before we go into that I would like to finish the saga of Turkish and other frontiers until we got back to the EU and these problems were over.

Leaving the north for the return ferry to Turkey was almost as bad as coming out, but at least it was daylight and we knew the form enough to expect the difficulties. An extra unscheduled problem was that Turkish shipping was helping the rescue operation in the Israeli-Lebanese fighting raging at the time and the previous day the ship had been cancelled. As a result they were very busy our day and my car had to go on a separate ship from the usual ferry. It was worrying sailing on a different vessel from my car, which had all our belongings and, although they left within a few minutes of each other, the boat with the cars arrived at a different port twenty minutes' drive away. Things became worse on arrival in Tasacu. I met up with a couple of Turkish car drivers who spoke little English but were determined to help us through. We negotiated the first port without too much trouble and were then bussed to the other where we saw our car vessel come in. There we went together round the series of offices until we came to a customs office which was closed. The customs officers had forgotten to come and we just waited calmly for about a half hour until a pair turned up and started on the paper work, filling in a pointless form, this time by hand and giving us a copy to surrender when we left Turkey. Our new friends at last smilingly told us all was done and we were all free to go, when we and they were hauled into yet another office to queue for a stamp or signature. After this again they were all smiles but unfortunately this had to be repeated one last time, and after about three hours we were finally on our way.

You may think this sounds bad but this was only a taster of what was to come. A few days later Wendy flew home from Istanbul and Rod came out to join me for six days. Surprisingly Attaturk airport was comfortable and efficiently run. The real trouble started when we crossed the border from Turkey to Bulgaria, which took five hours. It began when we eventually reached the Turkish customs office, where the customs officer found there was a missing stamp or signature on my passport or customs receipt. He did not know what to do so he sent me to the neighbouring booth where the other officer did not know either. After a great deal of pondering, he sent me to a back office which we had been to some time ago. Someone else said it was the wrong office, another looked at my passport and said there was no problem, and a coach driver pointed to an office about half a mile away behind which he thought I had to report. During all this time Rod was driving in the very slow queue for the border. We decided to be hopeful, but when we reached the border the missing stamp or signature mattered and we were not allowed through. They sent us back but the only helpful thing they did was to detail a young uniformed policeman to come in the car and guide us around. He took us to the place a half-mile back where eventually he found a more senior man who seemed to know something about it. He hardly spoke English but the problem seemed to be that an official at Tasacu had failed to put the right stamp on my passport; I suppose this could be associated with the notion that he had been called away from his supper to open the office. Although this new senior official saw the problem, he had no idea of the solution. He made a phone call and told us someone would return the call in ten minutes. In fact there were several calls at about ten minute intervals resulting in an apparently even more senior officer being called who examined my poor worn out and over stamped passport and we thought we would be on our way. This was one in a succession of false hopes because then the young policeman escorted us further back into Turkey for someone else to examine the papers and passport following which we did a U turn and went in a series back to each of the offices in turn for more signatures and stamps, each time our young but friendly policeman having to search for the right man. Nearly all these interviews were conducted with smoke being blown in my face. After this we reached the border for the second and last time, the interval between visits being one and a quarter hours.

There was then about an hour's wait to cross into Bulgaria, seemingly because few of the available booths on the Bulgarian side were open. What contmept for travellers customs officials have. Have you noticed when queing at immigration at airports how many booths are closed?

Crossing from Bulgaria to Romania by comparison presented little problems, just the inevitable passport stamping and a study of the Vehicle Registration Document. Going from Romania to Serbia was easy but this time instead of looking at the Vehicle Registration Document, by way of a change the officer wanted the Green Card. Going from there into Croatia, a glance at the passports was sufficient with no stamps and the same applied to Slovenia.

I wondered about this obsession with stamping passports in the south, especially in Turkey where at each crossing it is done several times. As far as I remember every official we saw was a man and I thought it may be that masturbation is a taboo and stamping documents combined with chain smoking is the nearest they can get to an acceptable substitute. This notion was confirmed at the Bulgarian-Romanian border where, attached to the officials' belts and hanging down near their flies, were rubber stamps with enormous red knobs on.

To sum up, based on my encounters, the Turkish officials are incompetent, rude, lazy and cruel. They are incompetent because they are working a system with no apparent order, making their own citizens as well as tourists go round in circles and waste a lot of time. They clearly have not been more than perfunctorily trained.

They are rude in that they never smile, smoke in your face and when faced with a problem they should but cannot solve they send you away on a pointless journey.

They are lazy because, apart from not bothering to turn up on one occasion, when faced with a problem they make no attempt to look after the punter and find out what to do.

They are cruel, not maliciously so, but because of the above faults they are not able to take on board how much unnecessary distress is caused and their only care is that you should get out of their way and stew in your own juice.

I have no idea if treating people like this, either their own citizens, foreigners or both, is a breach of human rights but if so I hope the EU authorities make sure this is corrected before further consideration is given to Turkey's entry. At present I imagine these frontiers, although not dangerous are almost as unpleasant as crossing a border from East to West in the height of the Cold War. I hope there cannot be anybody in any existing EU government who finds this sort of behaviour to any citizens, let alone EU citizens, acceptable.

Let's look at Turkey apart from the frontiers. In almost every respect Turkey is neither this nor that. It is certainly not first world, nor by any means third so I suppose it must be second world. I have not come across this concept before. It is similar to car insurance in that we all know whom the first and third parties are but who is the second? Apart from the large international ones, although the hotels seem to have friendly staff usually none of them speak English. The bedrooms are often small and dark although the plumbing works. The bath towels are likely to be smaller then a handkerchief.

We stayed in Side and Tasacu, both sea-side resorts on the south coast. Neither place was where foreign tourists went so we had no idea what it would be like putting up in a more international place.

We were placed by our agent in family hotels and the families seemed to be having a good time as they do if they like that sort of thing.

We then drove to Konya, a big town inland, where we could not find the hotel, as Gladys did not join us in Eastern Europe, Greece or Turkey. Not having a common language, the only way we managed was for Wendy to get into a taxi and for me to follow it. Konya was quite different from the sea area. As is well-known, Turkey is a Muslim but secular country and religion was much more in evidence here with most of the women wearing traditional dress. We had lunch at our hotel and I noted it did not serve alcohol; I had a horrible feeling that the town was dry. Fortunately later in the afternoon we were in a café in gardens in the centre of the city where I met a patient of my practice and he directed me to a wine-serving restaurant where we arranged dinner. The families were drinking tea from enormous ornate traditional silver pots.

Next we drove to Ankara for a night and stayed in the Sheraton and again I had to follow Wendy in a taxi. Security at the Sheraton was a bit of a poser. As we had seen the previous year in Istanbul, they examined the underside of vehicles with mirrors attached to poles, looking like giant versions of dentists' mirrors. As we drove through

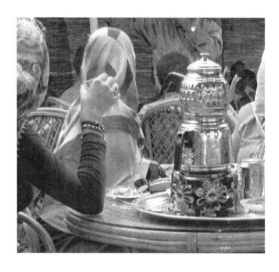

the hotel gates, the security staff examined Wendy's taxi and then my car with these instruments. The trouble was that as far as I could tell they would be able to see only the periphery of the underside of the cars and coaches. When we returned to the hotel by taxi in the evening the security staff had knocked off or taken a rest and there were no mirror wielders in evidence. This inconsistency cannot be lost on terrorists. The authorities must know this and it makes me wonder if, while realizing these precautions are useless, they need to put on some sort of show to reassure the customers. Once I start thinking in this way, I can start feeling negative about all security precautions and find it difficult to know when to stop. For example, we are ordered to switch off mobile phones in planes but no effort is made to see that we comply with this order, relying on our goodwill to stop the plane being diverted to a mountain top. They used to try this mobile phone rule nonsense in hospitals until patients and relatives noticed that all the staff, including the surgeons ignored it, breaking off from the consultation to answer their wives' calls about where they should have dinner that night.

I liked Ankara because it had a type of buzz to it. It was also a religious sort of place but not as much as Konya. In Konya hardly anyone spoke English but at least in Ankara they did in the hotel and restaurant. Wendy had her hair done in a busy shopping area and it was interesting walking around looking at the local scene. Backgammon seemed popular and in the open air cafes there were pairs of men complete with pairs of cigarette packets intent on the game. We had just learnt to play for this holiday and I tried to watch but I could not keep up with the speed of it. I did not see women play it. I was still surprised by the smoking. It looked as if every customer in every restaurant and café was at it and as you walked through the streets you walked through dog ends like autumn leaves in October.

After Ankara there was Istanbul, and as we had been here before we knew what to expect and allowed ourselves two nights here, even though I was not seeing a doctor. Istanbul is one of the most beautiful cities I know and a lot of fun. Many people speak English but if you ask them the way to anywhere it always seems to be through their shop. This is usually said with a twinkle in the eye. This work is not a specific travel guide but I will mention the Spice Bazaar where the spices are beautifully displayed and it has an excellent restaurant for lunch. If you like bargaining the Grand Bazaar is a worth a visit as it seems to have everything, including jewellers, electrical goods and clothes.

Although I like the Grand Bazaar, I am afraid bargaining is lost on me. When I see friends thrilled to have got something knocked off the price, I am concerned that they are so dazzled by what they did that they have not grasped what really happened. I assume that the shopkeeper or stall holder knows exactly what the retail price is that he needs to make his profit. Because of the culture of bargaining he has to add a considerable amount to allow the punter to persuade him to knock some off. Assuming, as I do, that few shoppers persist the whole way in every bargaining transaction, that means that most people are going to get ripped off to a certain extent some of the time. If the price was fixed as in Tesco or Sainsburys, shopping may be less fun but it would be cheaper.

I must not forget that this section is about Cyprus and it seems to have taken a long time to get there, metaphorically as well as literally. It is time to move on so I will not dwell very long on Cyprus.

We were relieved to find we had no trouble crossing the border into main Cyprus. For reasons known only to her the customs officer asked me to unpack the boot completely, but when I showed her my official letter from the Ministry of Health she called her boss and they smilingly waved me through. There were no difficulties on the drive back to the north.

We had dinner at a restaurant recommended by the hotel. It was as Alan Bennett once said in a different and ruder context, respectable but not remarkable. We have not worked out if taking advice from hotels on where to have dinner is a good thing to do because the results vary enormously. I have not yet determined if the concierge or receptionist gets a 'drink' from the restaurant or if the recommendation is because they genuinely believe it is good. In the end I suppose it could be one or the other. Still with nothing else to go on, this is often the way we choose our restaurants.

59

The next day I went to see the GP recommended by the Minister and she, Dr Elli Angelidou, worked in a welcoming health centre. We had a useful interview at the time but in the evening she and her daughter picked us up, showed us some of Nicosia, and then took us to a restaurant that they knew, where we had the most wonderful mezze. The food kept coming and each dish was special. Every time I think of it, I recall the flavour of one of the roast lamb dishes and I hope it will always remain unforgettable. Afterwards we saw more of the city and were told something of its history.

Slovenia

As well as driving a long way with Wendy to get to Cyprus, I, first with Wendy and then Rod, had to come a long way back before re-entering the EU, which we did at Slovenia. In the meantime we stayed one night each in Sofia, the capital of Bulgaria, Bucharest, the capital of Romania, Belgrade, the capital of Serbia and Zagreb, that of Croatia. Obviously we did not have time to see much en route but were conscious of some of the history through which we were travelling, much of it in my life time.

As I have described, we did not cross into Bulgaria until nearly midnight, reaching Sofia at five in the morning, where Rod found a taxi which I followed to our hotel. After a short sleep we made for Romania so we had hardly any impression of Sofia or indeed even of Bulgaria. We drove through Romania by day and thought it a lovely country. It appeared poorer than Bulgaria and there were lots of horse-drawn carts in the countryside. Everywhere we went, both in the town and country, the people seemed pleased to see us and anxious to help. Bucharest is an interesting place. There are long lengths of high jerry-built-looking residential concrete buildings so typical of Eastern Europe from communist times. Although ugly and squalid, it is possible they were necessary to get the population out of slums or overcrowding, into their own homes as quickly as possible after the second world war. The centre of the city is dominated by an enormous parliament building behind a vast piazza of large numbers of fountains. Although magnificent in scale, it is all rather spoilt by having been made of shoddy looking materials. It was all built in Ceausescu's time and I did not really discover what the population thought about it. They seemed to accept it because it was there.

We arrived in Bucharest on a Friday evening, when I had been away for exactly six weeks, so this was the half way mark. I took Rod out to what was recommended as a good restaurant and we started with champagne and then had a remarkably good meal here, with plenty of fresh vegetables and local meat, Rod having bear ragout.

Sometimes when one overdoes it, not even Eastern Europe is cheap but I must say the Romanians did us proud.

We crossed from Romania to Serbia over a long bridge across the Danube and the first thing we noticed was the scenery. The road was narrow but at first went along the river which was wide and then through tall hills, with a variety of majestic green trees on the right making an unforgettable lovely picture. After leaving the river the countryside stayed pretty, although the road was windy and slow. Belgrade is a large city, looking more prosperous than expected with a few usual sites like a striking cathedral and a national theatre. The hotel we stayed in was a Best Western and all I can say is it was not the best Best Western I have slept in. It was a similar experience to a no-frills airline where there was a big bruiser in a tee shirt to check us in and no one to manage garaging the car or even to take my cases in. Rod was not fazed by this but it is not my scene. I am out of place in Ikea and DIY shops. I once went to buy a toy kitchen range for my two year old granddaughter at "Toys Я Us" and when I chose it they told me to take it home on my 'motor' or they would deliver it for £15. At this point I left and went to John Lewis and chose something similar for the same price and had no difficulty in arranging free delivery. Although I do go on no-frills airlines such as Easy Jet or Ryanair, I accept now I am really a frills person.

The next day we drove from Belgrade to Zagreb. In Belgrade, the car was stopped by a policeman, seemingly at random. He examined the papers, and returned then to me with barely a word, much less any explanation of why he'd stopped us in the first place. It was a bit unsettling. We intended to add to our list of countries by popping over the border and having lunch in Bosnia but we spotted a large queue at the frontier and we were still phobic about this sort of thing. Although I am not conversant with the politics I could not help remembering that these countries were all part of Yugoslavia and that even though this country had to split up into smaller units, a little more maturity might have spared them these seemingly pointless barriers wasting their populations' time. When Ireland split off leaving Ulster and much bitterness on both sides they managed to keep their separate countries without obvious frontiers.

In Zagreb, Rod managed to navigate to our hotel, which was a Sheraton. Unfortunately it was the wrong one and although not full would not let us stay there at the agreed price. Eventually we found the right one, more at the edge of town. Without asking, we were upgraded to magnificent bedrooms. They were enormous and also full of luxuries. This was a real slice of luck because it is not the sort of room that I could afford.

I suppose with bedrooms you usually get what you pay for. I used to run on the theory that most of the time I was in a hotel bedroom I was asleep and therefore unaware of the surroundings and it seemed a waste of money to pay more than the minimum necessary for a good night's sleep. However, as we have got older we seem to want better and bigger rooms, but it is not clear what old age has to do with it. There are however some issues which, while being minor, seem important at the time. One of these is hangers. Most hotels offer hangers of varying quality but usually with a device so that the hook cannot be removed. This is insulting to clients who do not like it to be assumed that they are thieves. The cost of hangers compared with the room price is surely low enough that the hotel can bear the loss of those stolen. If not, I imagine that guests would find it easier to use wire hangers provided free by dry cleaning shops, which would spare them the unraveling of a Chinese puzzle when unpacking at the end of a long day.

There are just a couple of more minor grievances. Some hotels, it seems, especially in Italy, provide squares of small sheeting with no toweling material attached to dry faces and hands. It is not clear why they do this. I bet the money is not worth saving and I bet they have fluff on their hand towels at home. I must admit I discussed this with another man on holiday in Sicily recently and he said he preferred these as, when he shaves bits of toweling don't get stuck to his whiskers. This is a problem I have never noticed.

Another peculiarity that is worth mentioning is the eccentric variation of bedroom lighting. Sometimes it is minimalist, making the room seem dim and appear drab. Other rooms, even luxurious ones, have plenty of lights but none near the comfy chair where I want to read. The nonsense from which every traveller must have suffered is not knowing which switches are for which light. I usually tuck down later than Wendy and when I want to switch off the reading light I have to choose from the bank of switches by my side. When I get it wrong, instead of darkening the room, the main lights go on or the other side bed light goes on. One night when I switched off my light to go to sleep one table light remained alight on the other side of the room. I tried every wall switch but no luck. There was no pear switch on the wire and I wanted to achieve darkness without ringing down to the receptionist. Finally after several minutes I found a small white switch on the base.

Bathrooms are of course a bigger adventure than bedrooms. Wendy dislikes showers so we usually get one with a bath. I am taller than her and am sometimes forced to have a shower anyway. The variation of the tap and plug system is advancing at such a rate that it is almost becoming rocket science. Sometimes I just look at the knobs for a few minutes just to see what the tricks are. The most annoying is on turning any knob water comes from the showerhead all over my dry clothes. I have learnt that this cannot always be predicted and it is wise to turn the first tap very gingerly. Sometimes there are mixer taps with separate knobs, others one knob for both, with a separate one that appears to be the other but is really to control the temperature. Plugs are a law of their own although not usually dangerous. I dislike the ones that should be attached to broken chains, but the ones in situ where again a knob has to be turned can pose a problem as to which way it should go. Some of these leak and the water has to be kept running, having a disastrous effect on the ecology.

In the five star hotel in Tasaku in Turkey where we stayed three nights, plugs we're not provided in the baths or basins. On enquiry we were told they were not normal in that country but there was no explanation as to why large, inviting-looking bathtubs were installed.

The most interesting combination was the luxury bathroom in our room in the Sheraton in Ankara. Firstly, there was no plug in the basin so we could not wash our smalls. The bath was large but it had no hose of any sort so I had to have a shower to wash my hair. In the very smart shower cubicle, the hose was attached low down so I had to hold it throughout my shower. On the ceiling of the cubicle was a very large flat shower spray which was effective for my shampoo. However, it was obvious that when I pulled the button on the hose to get the water on to my hair I would be showered with a jet of the stinging cold water that was lurking in the intermediate pipe and there was no avoiding it. This proved to be the case.

Bathroom mirrors are usually OK in posh hotels but in pubs and bed-and-breakfasts there can be problems. Where the bathroom conversion has been done personally by a landlord who happens to be a short gentleman the mirror can be placed hopelessly low, especially for a tall man like myself. I find I have a choice of shaving while kneeling or depilating my belly button.

I usually need a pee during the night and it takes a few minutes to remember where the bathroom is and prepare a route in the dark. In the bathroom I use a torch because often the bathroom light switch is outside the door and I want to avoid a flood of light which might wake Wendy, and I object to peeing sitting down. I am surprised how few men I have spoken to use torches and I have no idea how they manage.

This reminds me of a common problem in English hotel bathrooms, especially small hotels and bed-and-breakfasts. This is the falling lavatory seat. It just will not stay up. Although it is possible to pee while aiming your willie with one hand while holding the seat up with the other, there is likely to be some missed spray, which is rather hard on the cleaning staff.

One new feature, or at least it is to me, is the change of provision of soap in some hotels. Instead of a tablet of wrapped soap by the basin, there is a device familiar to milk maids but useless to the rest of us. It is like an enormous teat and if you are strong enough to squeeze hard, or better still have learnt how to milk, there is a chance of getting some liquid mush out which serves for soap. There is a similar container on the wall at the side of the bath, just out of reach of the bather as it is hoped it will serve the showerer as well. Our Zagreb Sheraton did not suffer from this.

Anyway, after we checked in, we went into the city for dinner. We found what seemed to be a good restaurant. I looked at the menu and saw there was goose on the menu, one of my favourite dishes. Rod and I started on the wine and I looked forward to ordering the food, but when the waitress came she said the goose was off. I cannot remember if it had gone bad or run out – not escaped – just used up. It is often puzzling to know what 'off' means under these circumstances. In fact, with this problem, waiters are often lost for words. In Italy the favourite term is 'finished' and this, taken literally, seems unlikely if I am dining early. I suspect that in many restaurants 'finished' (in any language) is a euphemism for not started.

I was disappointed but relieved on looking again at the menu to find duck and in Croatia I knew it would be proper duck, not the Maigret nonsense. I was very angry when I was told that was no more of this either. Rod said I should not be cross with the waitress as it was not her fault. This statement at first seemed so obvious that I was quite taken aback at my manner, which was almost rude. On reflection, I wondered if he is right. The waitress was the representative of the establishment dealing with me, so surely it was her task to bear the brunt of the anger her establishment caused. I can see it both ways now but there is no doubt she should have told us the goose and duck were off when she gave us the menus.

It is annoying when dishes are unavailable. I know many times the chef cannot help it in that, when only fresh ingredients are used he can cook only so many portions, and will exhaust his supply if the demand for a particular dish is heavy. The problem would matter less if we were told on being handed the menu.

At last, we arrived at Ljubljana, the capital of Slovenia. Although this was part of the former Yugoslavia it seems more fitted to Western Europe and is now in the EU, sandwiched between Austria and Italy. It seems one of the more advanced new EU countries in that it adopted the Euro in 2007. Standing on the small bridges over the narrow river in Ljubljana, the capital made me think it was like a little Swiss town without the chalets.

We arrived in Ljubljana one evening and the next day Rod took the car to see the countryside while I walked round the town having a brief exploration before my appointment in the afternoon. Dr Nena Gucek was the GP I had planned to see and she had made it clear in advance that she was very busy and had little time. It took a lot of persuasion by email to get her to agree to see me. Consequently I was more nervous than usual and not hungry for lunch. I found a McDonalds, somewhere I had not eaten since my children were small. They were offering some sort of Chili Hamburger which looked more appetizing then most. I am afraid it was a disappointment, tasting just like their traditional food merely with a little chili wrapped round it. I remember about forty years ago my son and I split into opposite camps, he preferring Burger King while I went for McDonalds. My reasons were that as well as the latter having, in my view, nicer chips, the bun in the former always collapsed, leaving some sort of sick all over my hands with the risk of getting it on my clothes. Anyway, I washed carefully in the restaurant washroom having gained admission with some difficulty. The door was locked and to open it you needed a code printed on the receipt which of course I had not kept. Fortunately the waitress/hostess/server was kind and gave me the number.

Talking of public washrooms, finding the right door is getting harder as I am getting older. In my youth in England they used to say 'Gentlemen' or 'Ladies'. Then there was a big change to pictures, which seems sensible, especially with both multi-culturism and tourism. The pictures used to be the same, with the man wearing trousers and the woman a skirt where the sides stood out, to remove any doubt. Although women rarely wear anything other than trousers, it has obviously been impossible to remove this distinction but some artists, thinking the original drawings old-fashioned, have done new ones where it is becoming increasingly difficult to distinguish them. I have not yet gone into a 'Ladies' by mistake but I often have to spend longer studying the pictures to decide which the right one is. Occasionally I have waited to see who comes out of which and if there has been no one around have gone very gingerly into that which seemed more likely to be the 'Gentlemens' to see if there were urinals inside.

In England, where sometimes words are still used, it is interesting to note the change of terminology with time. 'Ladies' and 'Gentlemen' fell years ago to class consciousness and were replaced with 'Women' and 'Men'. I cannot understand why this classification has become unacceptable and given way to 'Female' and 'Male', as though we are no longer human but biological specimens. Either that or it is hoped that dogs and cats are going to learn to read and will be able to find the right door when house-trained.

Anyway, after lunch I saw Dr Gucek and it is fair to say I came away with the impression that she and perhaps most Slovenian GPs were the busiest in Europe, working under the most pressure I had seen since I left home.

In the evening we fancied a Chinese meal as a change from Balkan cooking. We both like Chinese food and the restaurant we found was fairly standard.

I seem to have written much about Slovenia for such a small country but once I get on to hotels and eating I always have a lot to say.

Hungary

Sadly, the day we came to Hungary it was cloudy and raining all the time so we may not have had a fair impression. This was Rod's last day, as late in the afternoon I was due to swap him for Wendy at Budapest.

Apart from being agricultural, the country seemed rather featureless until we came to Lake Balaton, which seemed as large as one of the major Swiss Lakes. Where we were there was no sandy beach, just some anglers. However it lacked the majestic snow-capped Swiss mountains and surprisingly we saw no sign of lake steamers.

We went from Lake Balaton to the airport. It was quite an experience. According to the map we had to drive up from the south to the airport on the way to the city. The airport was on a road parallel to ours, coming from a slightly more south easterly direction, and according to the map a new road from ours to the airport road was being built. Anyway, there was no evidence of it, so we had to drive more towards the city and were happy to find a sign for the airport which we followed. Unfortunately, that was the last for several junctions until we were nearly in town, now north of it and following the map when we saw one more sign then nothing. We had to ask at every garage until we were almost there. There are two terminals on different roads, about a ten minute drive from each other. They were signed Terminal One and Terminal Two but there was no hint of which was the domestic or international one. As you would expect, we chose the wrong one first and Rod began to be agitated he was going to miss his flight.

Why do authorities treat people like this? Have Hungarian road or airport magnates not been told by their friends that it is difficult to find their way out of Hungary? Is it plain incompetence or just a hangover from Soviet times, when it was normal to make leaving difficult, the idea being that no one would wish to leave a communist paradise?

Anyway Rod did catch his flight and after only a short wait, a lovely smiling Wendy appeared from the same plane and we found our hotel by the Danube, on the Buda side, without too much difficulty.

Budapest is a city worth visiting. As everyone knows, the Danube is a prominent feature, separating Buda from Pest and crossed by an interesting group of bridges. Looking down from the Fisherman's Bastion on the hillside of Buda across the Danube to the parliament building in Pest gives a quick, unforgettable feeling of the majesty of the place.

My appointment next morning, a Thursday, was with Dr Vilmos Dani whom, as he worked in the afternoon on that day, I saw at home. He is a keen sportsman and is the doctor to the Hungarian equivalent of our Lawn Tennis Association, and he looked superbly fit. His house was beautifully decorated and, like the other doctors' homes I visited, very comfortable but not opulent.

Slovakia

Our next destination was Bratislava, the capital of Slovakia. Although it is only a short drive from Budapest, Wendy took over the driving and I had a sleep. Wendy woke me to tell me she had driven into the wrong country, having found herself in Austria. Based on the study of a sample of one, many years ago I founded a law which states that the quality of a person's navigation is in inverse proportion to their cooking and Wendy is one of the world's best cooks. I discovered that the law was not universal when my daughters grew up. To be fair, the different frontiers are so close to each other that it was not a big problem to get into the wrong nation. The frontiers in this region are all adult and civilised.

Slovakia has the reputation of being the poor relation of the old Czechoslovakia but superficial inspection does not confirm this. The towns are teeming with new cars and there was much building in Bratislava. This is a typical old ex-Warsaw Pact capital with enormous concrete tower blocks in the suburbs while in the centre are a whole succession of small medieval and enlightenment period squares, with many beautiful buildings of varied architecture and a lot of history to see. It seems to be the stag party capital of Europe at present, especially for English celebrants.

It was difficult to find the part of town where the Presidential Palace was, our hotel, the Crowne Plaza being nearby. Gladys, of course, did not work here. Just before Wendy found a taxi she asked a customer at a filling station. He did not speak English but Wendy showed him on the map what she wanted. It was obviously in a different part of the city but he indicated that he was going there and we should follow him, and he kept us in his mirror the whole way. This is one of these acts of kindness that travellers get which are unexpected but always such a pleasure to receive. One of the advantages of Eastern Europe is that not only are top hotels more affordable but they, unasked, give generous upgrades. We had a suite with a separate bathroom, shower room, lounge with business desk and two televisions (why two?) and a bedroom.

The next day, a Saturday, I had my appointment with Dr Tibor Hlavatý. He works in what was one of the old communist country polyclinics and it was very large. It appeared to be attached to a hospital. When I arrived by taxi a little early, it was almost deserted. The janitor, who spoke no English, let me in but had no clue why I was there. He recognized the name Dr Hlavatý and bade me sit while he went to make a phone call. I began to get a horrible feeling that there was some mistake and all my future plans would go awry. It was a relief after a few minutes to see that I need not have worried and he turned up expecting me and pleased to see me. He was so friendly that he asked me to have lunch with him at a nearby restaurant. I would normally have been thrilled at this, and did in fact accept. My problem was that my younger daughter, Victoria, had flown out to Bratislava for the day to see us and obviously I wanted to lunch with her. Unlike Wendy, I had seen none of my children for more than six weeks and it would be another five weeks before I arrived home.

We had a fascinating conversation over lunch all about life in Czechoslovakia before Perestroika, but I was conscious of the pull to get to my family. After a foreshortened meal, I arrived at the square only to find that, not expecting me so soon, they had signed up for a guided walking tour of the old city and were part of a very small group. The guide, a lovely lady who clearly knew her job, seemed to go on forever and all the time I was more trying to talk to Victoria than listen and it was a relief when it finished. It is no surprise that I remember very little of the history of the city but that it used to have a different name.

It was wonderful spending the rest of the afternoon with Victoria before she had to leave for the airport. She had a long day, having had to wake up at four o'clock that morning. Later, Wendy discovered that the hotel had given her vouchers for us to have a free drink in the bar and a free five course dinner. At the time she had no idea of the reason for this generosity but we enjoyed the drinks. When we went into dinner, we were almost the only customers although we were there at a normal time. The dining room was large, white and luxurious. I cannot say there was anything wrong with the food but after two of the five courses we could eat no more and were very embarrassed when the waiter brought a heaving plate of meat and vegetables, none of which we could touch. I cannot remember what we had ordered. Wendy thought we had filled up on the first courses but I think it was something I cannot define about hotel food.

Unless a hotel has a special restaurant, we almost never eat in hotel dining rooms but choose local restaurants. We are not the only ones because I have noticed when travelling that often hotels have sumptuous dining rooms and yet these seem to be empty. This emptiness makes them look unattractive and presumably is the reason why hotels give free vouchers. There is such a thing as a free dinner therefore but it is often best avoided.

Talking about food again reminds me of water and of course the old vexed question of tap or bottled. Obviously there is nothing to discuss if you prefer sparkling water but my choice is still. When I was a child in the forties my parents ordered only Evian water in France, thinking tap water was not safe. The British were very chauvinistic immediately after the war, and for all I know, before it also. It was strange therefore that the UK was fined by what was the EEC many years ago because our tap water did not meet European standards. Unless you are highly neurotic, or are unable to understand evidence, you are likely to agree that the choice is no longer a matter of safety but just taste. Friends who buy bottled water tell me they find it tastes better. There seems no possibility of their putting this idea to a blind tasting. I would like to pour out a certain number of glasses of tap water (I would ask a statistician how many) and an equal number containing their chosen bottled water at identical temperatures into glasses with coded labels and see if they can tell the difference. They would need to gain a sufficient score to demonstrate that they can truly tell the difference. Just getting two out of two correct could just be chance. As I would want to be seen to be unprejudiced like the punter, I would not know the code. This would be known only by an agreed moderator.

This idea is the basis of evidence-based prescribing. It is known as a 'double blind trial'. I mentioned these at the beginning but the concept is so important and basic that it is worth going over it again. When there is a new drug whose makers claim does things better than previous drugs, it is put to a similar test. After all tests possible for safety, followed by permission from a local ethical committee, the drug, usually a tablet, is administered to a large number of people and an identical tablet, which could be a dummy tablet known as a placebo, is given at random to an identical number of people who are similar in age and as far as possible medical condition. All the patients involved are counselled and give fully informed consent for this. Sometimes, instead of a placebo, an active drug is used which the pharmaceutical company claims their new one is superseding. The doctors or nurses both administrating the tablets and measuring the effects are not informed which patients are taking what. These experiments are known therefore quite reasonably as 'double blind trials' and to most doctors and certainly to me are the gold standard of assessing what works best.

Anyway, if it is used for medication and can be used for water there is no stopping the notion. As is well-known, there is significant concern about obesity at present. Many people drink refreshing fizzy beverages such as Coca-Cola and Pepsi-Cola. I have noticed that few children and only some adults go for the sugar free options. By not doing this they are taking in many pointless and, in a lot of people, harmful calories. Occasionally I have asked why they do this and the answer is that they prefer the taste. It may seem arrogant for me to question the idea that they know what they like but still, I wonder if they really can tell the difference. I would love to see a double blind trial done on the subject and if there is no significant difference either in discrimination of taste or preference, it would be reasonable to ask the manufacturers to concentrate their marketing on the sugar-free drinks.

What about cooking and gardening? Could the principles of the 'double blind trial' be applied to them? How much do television presenters of these topics depend on evidence, how much is good experience and how much is nonsense? For example, many recipes advise sea salt. Apart from the romantic-sounding name, this, like table salt, is sodium chloride, nothing more or less except of course more money. It is obvious therefore once it is put into the cooking the final dish cannot taste any different whichever salt is chosen. I do accept that cooking and gardening are arts as well as sciences and therefore more licence should be allowed for fatuous advice, but it would do no harm if the readers of instructions and recipes made some attempt to consider the validity of the information.

I know nothing about horticulture but once bought from the local gardening centre a Yucca for my study. Unfortunately it did not thrive. The shopman told me never to add fertilizer or any chemicals. Wendy told me I was not watering it enough while her sister said I should water it infrequently. I went back to the shop and a different assistant said it was my fault entirely in that I was not adding the appropriate nutrients which he then sold me. What was obvious was that not only did none of my advisers know what to do but they did not know that they did not know and were therefore willing to give useless advice. I realize now that science should have been brought into this art of growing indoor plants and if I had contacted a faculty of horticulture in a University, someone could have found the answers from double blind trials published in peer-reviewed journals.

I am afraid that once on this train of thought there is no stopping of it, but I must say something about how science and art get mixed up in the word 'fresh'. When we were courting, around 1960, we would occasionally splash out (£3 at the time) for a meal at The Angus Steak House in Soho, which was a branch of a new chain. This was before the Trade Descriptions Act. They claimed that their meat was so fresh that it was 'rushed down overnight from Scotland'. We believed that and thought it great, as it was not for some years that we learnt that meat needs to be kept and hung for a period to get to its best. Eggs are another example of this. Cafes advertise 'fresh eggs' and as you taste them you think of the chicken sitting in a bed of straw with all the activities and smells of the farm yard around. In fact, although I admit I have not done the experiment, I would be surprised if anyone could identify a fresh egg over a two week old one (kept in a fridge) boiled and served under identical conditions. Talking of eggs, Rod and I, as mentioned earlier, spent many hours talking of the ethics of battery farming. Some people claim that eggs from free-range chickens taste better than those of battery farmed ones. Apparently it is something to do with the yolk. Again I would like to see evidence demonstrated for this ability to discriminate.

I think this flexibility with the truth is the stuff of art and adds to the enjoyment of eating. I do not agree however that there should be any flexibility in medicine. As advice which includes lifestyle changes, as well as medication and surgery, can have an adverse effect on the person's enjoyment of their life, it must never be given unless it can be shown to be true or as likely as possible to be so. For example, the evidence of the dangers of smoking is overwhelming and doctors have a duty to make sure every smoker has informed knowledge of this, but what about the five portions of fruit and vegetables a day? There is no doubt (providing that you are not living in an impoverished society) that fruit and vegetables are not good for you, although it is true that they are less bad than any other food. So to avoid or treat obesity or diabetes, as well as reducing your food intake, you will do less harm with fruit and veg than meat and butter; that is the best that can be said for them. The figure of five portions a day is balderdash and it is sad that it is taken seriously. It is true that there are protective chemicals in fruit and veg but not nearly enough to make any difference.

I will finish this subject with vitamins. Apart from very few people in some ethnic groups, or with very rare illnesses, nobody in western society will benefit from added vitamins. There is enough in the normal food intake and health does not improve by taking more. I shed a silent tear every time I see a customer walk through the doors of a health food shop. The older readers will remember tonics in their youth and realize now that the whole concept had been consigned to the dustbin. Incidentally, you can neither treat nor prevent colds with Vitamin C tablets.

Austria

Our next country was Austria and this time we found that we had entered the correct state. My contact doctor was Dr Waltraud Fink, a doctor whom I found on an academic website. She was the doctor I mentioned earlier who was a little hostile when I first approached her but when I explained what I wanted, she could not have been more helpful. In fact, she was so keen on the project that she invited us to stay with her and also thought I should see another Austrian GP so that I could have a more balanced picture. This resulted in her arranging for me to see a colleague in another part of the country. We therefore arrived at Dr Gustave Kamenski's house on the Sunday for lunch. His surgery is in his house. The family were wonderful hosts. Gustave took me into his consulting room to start our interview then we joined his family and Wendy for lunch. I think it may have been typically Austrian in that it started with spinach soup and was followed by lots of Wiener Schnitzels. Following that and the completion of our interview they drove us around the countryside to see a chapel, which Gustave's wife Brigitte had helped to renovate.

Because in a referendum they rejected nuclear power, and this was even before Chernobyl, there are wind farms everywhere, often dominating the countryside. We learnt that where we were, the wine industry is important and we passed numerous vineyards. Later we drove to Vienna and stayed overnight.

Next day we tried sight-seeing in the pouring rain. Because of this, we did not see much, but we had been there for a long weekend in 1980. It still seems worth seeing and we hope to go back. We had coffee in the opera house and they were playing Faust on a large screen, making us reluctant to leave.

In the afternoon we drove back into the countryside, this time on the other side of Vienna going towards the Czech Republic. We were on our way to Dr Fink's village. Gladys seemed to have difficulty finding the right house but this was not a problem because we found a pedestrian who spoke English and of course knew the local doctor and her house. When we arrived, she was out visiting a patient but her sister was there to greet us.

I must say I was rather nervous. I was afraid that Waltraud being so academic, would be formidable and I might be frightened of her. Also, as I will discuss when we come to the section on France, I have a fear of staying in other people's homes. However, we need not have worried. The sisters were kindness itself and when Waltraud came after a few minutes she was very easy to talk to. She is single and lives alone. She used to live in the same house as the surgery but now has her own home a few minutes away by car. Her sister lives nearby with her family and her husband is a farmer with a wine cellar. I began to wonder if viniculture was taught in school as a core subject in Austria.

The family make honey, wine and apricot schnapps. Wendy spent some time there, while Waltraud took me to her surgery

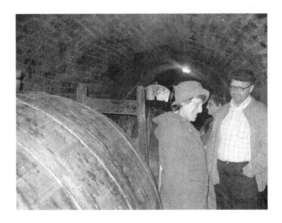

where I was allowed to sit in while she treated a patient and then we had our interview.

For supper we all met up in a large cellar, presumably a wine cellar, since unlimited wine kept coming. There were large platters of sandwiches with meat and cheese surrounded by cucumber and chilies. I set next to the brother-in-law who seemed like Mr. Wardle in the Pickwick Papers. He did not speak English nor I German but in spite of that we got on like a house on fire. Afterwards he took us to his cellar and it was a pleasure to see his pride and love of his bottles. It was a magical evening.

Back at Waltraud's house we had the guest bedroom and bathroom to ourselves and there was no embarrassment, so I had worried needlessly. Next morning Waltraud cooked us scrambled eggs and we were on our way to Prague.

The Czech Republic

I was sad when Czechoslovakia split in to two countries but I admit I knew nothing about the issues and that it was none of my business. What I cannot excuse is their lack of imagination to find a proper name for themselves; I always thought that it was here bohemians originated and they did not lack ideas.

Even without Gladys, here we had no difficulty in finding our hotel but the drive through the countryside was difficult because of roadworks and incompletely sign-posted diversions. You cannot blame only the Czechs for this because it happens everywhere, and is another example of how so many people, such as, in this case, the sign erector organizers and testers, including the people responsible for their selection, training and appraisal, are in the wrong job.

As is well-known, Prague is a beautiful city but I am sad to report that as a tourist attraction, through no fault of its own, it is rapidly losing it. Other equally beautiful cities such as Paris, Vienna or Budapest are just that, cities where the inhabitants go about their lives surrounded by historic and lovely surroundings and tourists mix with them and share this beauty. However, although Prague has everything the others have, including the Old Town Square, the castle, Charles Bridge and old Jewish quarter, the town is too small to accommodate the visitors. I had the impression that all the shops in the central area were for the tourists and not for the locals. There was an abundance of places to eat and drink and an excess of tat souvenir shops. It was almost as though we were visiting

Disneyworld rather than a capital city and like that the magic soon palls. I am not sure there is much that they can do about this, being a victim of their own success. They should not though have allowed the restaurants to spread into the main square, destroying some of its grandeur. It is still worth seeing but I would recommend if possible going mid-week out of season.

We stayed at the Corinthian Panorama Hotel on the edge and mostly went in and out of town by metro. I think by now I was staying in too many hotels because I was to phone my doctor, Bohumil Seifert, and make arrangements for him to pick me up from the hotel at four o'clock, take me to his surgery and then bring me back. When the time came he did not arrive so with sickening anxiety, anxiety because I knew an appointment had to fail some time and, if so, the whole project, I phoned him. It turned out that I had told him the wrong name of the hotel and he was at its branch elsewhere in town. Fortunately he still came and was friendly and happy to show me his practice.

Wendy fixed the dinner that night. As is her wont, she asked advice from the concierge and I suppose this was the right thing to do, in that this was quite an up market hotel so it could be hoped he knew what he was doing. This turned out to be the case in that we went by taxi to a restaurant just under the Charles Bridge with lovely views of it. It was also a fine meal with good service but I cannot remember what we ate. We had had goose the previous evening so it would be unlikely to have been that.

Germany

Driving to Berlin reminded me of so much history made in my life time. Firstly the Second World War and then the Cold War. Always when in Germany, as I am a Jew, I feel vaguely guilty, although never enough to stop me going. I am not sure if it is a sense of selfishness or whether it is a spirit of enquiry that if something has happened I want to see it, however much I disapprove of the morals. For example, in 1983, on my first visit to what was the Soviet Union, one of the first things we did was to queue up to see Stalin's body. In 1986 we did a weekend trip to West Berlin and were able to go by coach through Checkpoint Charlie for a brief look at the East. Our guide, while speaking perfect English, told me she had not seen West Berlin for twenty years. A few years ago, on a sight-seeing visit to Krakow, I left Wendy who did something more artistic, and took the excursion to Auschwitz. Because of the history of the place, I was humbled by the thought that comparing myself with my fellow Jews of sixty years ago I was so lucky to have been born where I was, both in history and geography. Compared with them I had plenty of food, could go into and out of Germany or Poland as I pleased, and had a full set of human rights, including freedom from fear of most things.

We drove past Dresden, which conjured up more thoughts and then to Berlin where our hotel was near the Brandenburg Gate. After checking in, we saw some of the local sights, apart from the Gate, and this included the new memorial to the murdered Jews of

Europe. I thought they had got this exactly right; it was both pleasing to look at and restful, providing a good environment in which to reflect on the events it was commemorating.

Berlin was one of the cities where friends were coming out to see us. This time we were blessed with two couples, Val and Geoff, and Hazel and Mervyn. Unfortunately they were delayed because of an Al-Qaeda plot to blow up more aircraft. This was the one which prevented passengers from carrying liquids for a period. However, they did come late that night and we were together next day. I saw my doctor, who was about a twenty minute taxi ride along a busy road into East Berlin. The road seemed to go on for ever, rather like the Edgware Road near where I live. I realized that owing to the war the buildings could not be old and when I looked at them this was obviously true. They were not beautiful either. The meeting was with Dr Andreas Kärsten, who was part of a small group practice. As ever, it was fascinating, and then I returned to the hotel the way I came. It is probably getting obvious by now that I enjoyed the interviews. Not only was each one a success, but they were all different and not one was anything but a pleasure. Even with the entire sight-seeing, our friends coming out, the food and drink, the interviews remained the best part.

On getting back to my room, I phoned Wendy who told me she had met up with the others and they were all about to have lunch near the Brandenburg Gate. I was excited to join them all as this was the first time we had seen friends since Rome about five weeks earlier. After lunch we all took an open bus tour which included many things, including a detailed look at Checkpoint Charlie. Although the history here was worth seeing, the whole area has become rather tacky, with plenty of silly souvenir stalls. In the evening, after champagne in our room we had dinner out of doors on the Unter Der Linden.

Poland

I had great difficulty in finding a doctor in Poland. Eventually I phoned a distinguished London professor who had written an article in the British Medical Journal (BMJ) He was very busy but listened long enough to understand the problem and he gave me the email address of a presumably equally distinguished professor in Warsaw. This led to a trail which finished in Krakow, where the professor there arranged for me to see a colleague, Dr Janusz Krzyszto . This caused me to change my schedule because I had not planned to visit Krakow, but the adjustments were not difficult. We arrived in Krakow on a Saturday afternoon, had a day off on the Sunday, I saw Dr Krzyszto on the Monday morning and then belted off to Warsaw to stay one night en route to Lithuania.

Our hotel in Krakow was easy to find with the telephone help of the hotel receptionist. It was near one of their two Tescos on the edge of town. The Tesco was enormous and appeared to be the biggest I had ever seen. I have no real opinion as to whether shops should be open on Sundays, or rather I have strong opinions but unfortunately they conflict; I do believe though if you are going to have Sunday opening you should do it properly and not force this six hour nonsense. Anyway this Tesco was open twenty four/seven to use the horrible expression popular now. I took advantage of this to get some replacement clothes, and on the Sunday morning I had my only hair cut of the trip.

There is something about having haircuts away from home. In the last few years I have preferred to shampoo my own and settle for a simple cut at a barber's shop. In the past I used to have it shampooed for me and tried barbers and ladies' salons. Sometimes I used so-called 'Unisex' shops but as far as I could make out these were merely ladies' salons that wanted to attract men's custom as well. The main difference was in the washing of the hair. In a man's shop, the customer bends his face forward over the basin, while in the woman's it is laid back looking up at the ceiling. No barber or stylist can tell me the reason for this and seem surprised to be asked but I wondered if it is associated with the missionary position for coitus.

Krakow has a large medieval square with much historical architecture. Not far is the Jewish quarter where there was a lot of Jewish history to be seen but it was not clear if there were many Jews who had survived and stayed. Most of the synagogues were museums. There was a splendid and popular restaurant which, while not being kosher, served traditional Jewish food and the cooking was unbelievable. I should say that it was just like the food Momma used to make, but my mother was born in London and her cooking was English traditional. Also in this Jewish quarter was an Indian restaurant and this may have seemed incongruous at first, until one remembers the history of London's East End, where Indians have moved into what was once the Jewish quarter. I used to be addicted to Indian food and would feel ill when my serum curry level fell below seventeen nanograms per litre. In the old days, after three weeks driving around France in our summer holidays, we used to drive straight from Dover to "The Raj Mahal" in Edgware for a Vindaloo fix before going home.

Dr Krzyszto arranged to collect me from the hotel and it was a treat coming down in the lift after breakfast to see a man holding a placard with my name on it just like being met by a mini-cab driver at an airport. He is a single-handed GP as is so common in Europe and like others he struck me as being rather lonely. Again like others he is not unhappy about this. Single-handed doctors here and abroad value their freedom to make their own decisions where those of us in group practices have to persuade our partners of our view and this is not always possible. Also there is no doubt that single-handed doctors have a much closer relationship with their patients. More details of these issues can be found in *The Medical Part*.

That evening we stayed in Warsaw as planned but it was only overnight, so apart from having another memorable dinner, goose again, the town this time left very little impression. Fortunately we had been here for a weekend in 2001. There were plenty of staff in all the restaurants in Poland, which rather surprised me. Many of the restaurants near where we live employ Eastern European waiters and waitresses from all the countries, and in 2005 when we went touring round Scotland, it seemed that for almost every meal we were served by Poles, leaving me with some anxiety that there would be none left to wait on us while we were in Poland.

Lithuania

Leaving Poland for Lithuania we had to go a long way round as the direct route went through Belarus and a visa was needed which frankly was not worth the expense or hassle. What is wrong with these people? I suppose it is still a police state that will be liberated from within one day, but meanwhile I have every sympathy for the inhabitants. Fortunately, Lithuania had all the appearances of a free country with no visas or any delay at the borders.

They seem to be spending plenty of EU money. The motorways in Lithuania are a little unusual in that left turns and u-turns are allowed and also there are bus stops. Apart from being places where buses presumably stop, it is hard to see the function because often there appears to be no sign of habitation and if anyone did anything so strange as to alight there, it is difficult to see where they would go.

The old town of Vilnius has, at present, almost entirely disappeared behind scaffolding and various other forms of wrapping, as it appears to be being totally renovated. There is a central square which could possibly be pretty but the whole of it is being re-laid and all one can hear is the sound of stone-cutting machines echoing within the endless barriers.

Another couple of close friends, Ruth and Ronnie, came to join us for our stay in Vilnius. The first night we had dinner in a pseudo-converted barn but it had excellent service and interesting food, although we did not have goose this time. The next day while I was at a doctor's clinic they and Wendy met an old friend who commuted between Belarus and Vilnius. He was bi- if not tri-lingual and knew all about the systems. Not surprisingly, he knew all the best restaurants and as we all fancied steak that day he took us to the best in town. It was a lovely evening so we sat outside, but as time went on it became increasingly colder. I wondered if this was a feature of Northern Europe because the staff were prepared for it and came out with a pile of blankets for us to wrap ourselves in.

Last Christmas, one of my sons-in-law bought me a heavy book on the history of the Jews since the seventeenth century. It was written by an orthodox rabbi from New York and it was history from his point of view. Briefly, he seemed to be saying that before the nineteenth century most Jews lived in Eastern Europe. (This really means the Ashkenazi Jews; the Sephardic Jews who were also orthodox lived more around the Mediterranean, had slightly different rituals and spoke Hebrew with different pronunciation.) In those days most of the Jews were religious and kept all the laws, including never breaking the Sabbath laws or eating food that was not strictly kosher. As always in religious groups, there were schisms, the main one being that one side, the Chassidim, thought more time should be spent communicating with the Almighty while the other, the Misognim thought that all right-thinking Jews should spend their free time studying the Jewish Law: in other words, the first five books of the Old Testament (the Torah).

Lithuania, along with Poland and Russia was one of the great centres of Jewish study and there were many famous rabbis there. It was in this country that yeshivas were first founded. These were schools devoted to teaching study of the Torah and very little else. Sadly, although of course I knew about the Holocaust and that most Lithuanian Jews had been murdered, I had had no knowledge of the rich vein of Jewish history there, so it all passed me by. It will be a good reason for going back though.

Latvia

On the surface, Latvia was similar to Lithuania and the capital Riga was another lovely Hanseatic town. Again we were joined by friends, Marilyn and Phillip this time, a couple who wanted to visit two cities and they joined us on the next drive to Estonia.

The hotel in Riga, the Monika Centrum was the first not to have our booking. However they were very nice about it, and recommended where we should have lunch nearby and afterwards gave us the presidential suite, with a bedroom with a four poster bed (Wendy loves this sort of thing), lounge and bathroom with separate lavatory. She thought this was the prettiest room so far, and they threw in free internet access.

On a Friday afternoon I left Wendy, Marilyn and Phillip and walked to a private clinic about a mile from the hotel. I had been unable to arrange to see a state doctor before leaving. Two young lady doctors who worked in this clinic arranged to see me. It turned out that they had both been trained by the same trainer, Dr Lasmanis who works in the national health. As a very kind gesture, they had invited him to the interview and he gave me much of my information.

It was lucky they did so, because, as well as working only in the private sector they had rather soft voices and I am getting a little deaf. Before coming away, I had acquired a pair of hearing aids. I have found them invaluable at practice meetings but on the whole I do not like wearing them. They make the whole world seem different and unreal. It has been explained to me that I am not used to having sound returned to normal and matters would improve if I wore them all the time. I am trying to do this.

Hearing aids do other funny things though. I am typing this on a computer and wearing them now and it sounds as though I am using a manual typewriter. My car, being rather large, is fitted with warning beepers front and back each end giving different notes. When I am wearing the hearing aids, it sounds as though there is a band of trumpeters in front and another of buglers behind. The worst shock though was when I had my first pee in a lavatory at home. When aiming for the water at the bottom of the pan, instead of hearing the usual splash, there was the sudden noise of a machine gun firing at me.

Estonia

We had first visited Tallinn on a Baltic cruise in 1997 and we thought it was a fairy-tale sort of place. It was the first time we had seen one of these lovely Eastern European towns. The guide told us then that they wanted to join the EU but there was a problem in that they had a large ethnic Russian population, who had not integrated and did not have full human rights. This was against EU rules. Well, as everyone knows, they eventually joined the EU and I assumed the problem was solved. However, I hear that at a meeting the Russian president was complaining that the Russians still do not have human rights in Estonia.

Since our previous visit, Tallinn has, unfortunately, like Prague, lost the plot. It is a beautiful old town, almost as pretty although on a smaller scale. There are many medieval Hanseatic buildings. What with the reputation for beauty combined with the fact that it is a port where big cruise ships come in, it has become overwhelmed by tourists. We were there on a Saturday evening where it was like Nottingham on a bad day. Crowds of young people swarmed around, some of the women remarkably scantily dressed and many people drunk. Certainly they did not appear interested in the beauty of the town, merely the fact that it was a cheap place to come and have a party. On the Sunday morning the old town was different; everywhere there were groups of older people following a guide holding a large umbrella. There were groups of Germans, English and also some Americans and Australians doing a Baltic Cruise. Although

Tallinn is a lovely old town, it is not enjoyable being there, and apart from a quick half day's glance at it I would counsel avoiding it for the time being except perhaps well out of the tourist season.

It seems there is a vicious circle in these old Eastern European towns in which Tallinn has been badly caught up. The Soviets left about fifteen years ago and people realized that they could now visit this lovely and interesting old town. As they came in increasing numbers, the tourist trade moved in to serve them with many souvenir shops, restaurants in fake old Estonian style and large hotel blocks, probably too many of the last. Then crowds of young people, many having stag or hen parties, started visiting as they heard there was a cheap place where tourist needs were catered for. Add a low cost airline and the goose is cooked. However, possibly because of the tourist trade, Estonians seemed to speak the most and best English of the three Baltic States.

Our hotel, the Reval Hotel Central, also did not have our booking but were most unpleasant and unapologetic about it. They gave us the impression that it was all our fault, even though we showed them written confirmation from the agent. Eventually, after making us wait for what seemed a long time in the reception area, they sorted it out but their attitude was a marker for the whole tone of the hotel. Anyway, we arrived on a Saturday and as my appointment with the doctor was not until the Monday, we were here for one of my few three night stays. This gave us a chance to unpack completely.

I like unpacking on holiday. As we saw earlier, the Michaels have never travelled light and amongst other luggage we have one large and one small suitcase each. The smaller is always used when away for short trips and the larger is not needed. Also, on long motoring journeys such as this one, only the smaller cases come into the hotel if we are staying only one night. My smaller case has had a lot of use because over the years I have been to many conferences and workshops. I like to use different gear when away and it stays permanently in the small case. Wendy swears this is my fantasy that the prime minister or a film star is going to get taken ill somewhere in the world and insist on sending for me, and therefore I keep my case packed and ready.

For reasons I cannot explain I have grown to love these possessions, I know the provenance of most of them and get exquisite pleasure from using them. In no particular order they include a beautifully made small torch I bought in Lyons in 2003, a pair of travel slippers in a pouch bought in a shopping mall in San Diego in 1991 (the pouch was thrown away by the steward on a ship between Korea and Japan in 1995 but I still use the slippers,) a wonderfully made shoe horn given by a patient who owns a posh West End men's shop, nail-cutters bought from a pharmacy in Krakow in 2001 and a global travel radio alarm clock given by my goddaughter for my recent birthday. I changed to shaving with a brush at the instigation of the above patient some years ago but still used brushless shaving cream anyway but did not like it. However my nephews bought me a kit with a brush, razor and a pot of shaving cream for the same birthday and this has joined the collection. I am very careful to check they are all packed each morning as the loss of any one of them would spoil the holiday.

We spent most of the weekend sight-seeing and on the Monday morning Wendy went off with our friends, while I went to see the doctor, Dr Sirje Linntam. After our interview, she walked back with me to the old town and showed me buildings I had not seen. Afterwards I was on my own for lunch. I found another curry house and thought I would have one for a change. The meal was different from the standard Bangladeshi you get at home; it was more like eating a curry in India. I asked the front-of-house lady where she came from but she was not friendly and did not want to talk about herself. I enjoyed the meal so much that next day after our friends had gone to the airport, I took Wendy there for lunch, before finding our ferry for Finland.

Finland

We took an afternoon ferry from Tallinn to Helsinki. In Finland almost the first thing to be noticed after having spent so much time in Eastern Europe was that there were no crowds of tourists and no longer the massed high rise cheap apartment blocks ubiquitous in former communist countries. In Poland once I saw a block of flats so long that there was more than one bus stop along the road at the side of it and a McDonald's in the middle.

Our hotel, a rather better Best Western, which had a sauna which we did not use, was sadly in the outer suburbs and to avoid missing the town we had to take an expensive taxi ride in. It was worth it just to see the cathedral and walk along the main road. It is unbelievable how we still found the main roads of each town different and exciting. After seeing the cathedral, we must have got to the wrong part because there were very few restaurants where we were and it took some time to find somewhere where we would like to eat, to us one of the most important events of the day, competing only with the interviews. We found a restaurant in an hotel and it had a very motherly waitress. For the first time, Wendy had reindeer meat. It did not surprise me that she chose it. In South Africa she was quite happy to eat ostrich. I always thought no new food would faze her. (Please understand although we are Jewish we are rather lax.) The only foods she will not eat are rabbit, which I understand, and tripe, which is my favourite but revolts her, all my family and most of my friends. I am not as fortunate as her in that something happened to me about the age of forty, when my eating choices became set in stone. Not only had I never eaten rabbit, but neither had I tried venison, ostrich, reindeer and many others of a similar nature. I am really stuck with about eight dishes including roast beef, pink roast lamb, steak or chops, fried plaice or poached salmon. There are a few others. I like duck but it must be ducky duck. In other words it has to taste of duck. A whole roast duck carved in front of us is fine. Breast of duck, or as it is in French menus Maigret de Canard, is an abomination. It is clearly made for diners who hate duck but are unable to admit it. It comes as attractive pink slices of tender meat with no taste at all, certainly not of duck. Sadly, since the old Caprice died in the 1960s, most restaurants have forgotten the proper taste of duck. As will be obvious by now, we like goose but fortunately it is rarely ponced about with and you usually get goosey goose.

Next day we left early for Turku on the west coast where our doctor was and he had arranged to pick me up from my hotel at half past eleven. Although Gladys works in Helsinki, she is not available on the road to Turku, so we had to find the hotel by navigation and asking. Now we were back in the west there was no difficulty in communicating. The doctor I was seeing, Mårten Kvist, was an academic found through WONCA. He was a professor of general practice; although no longer teaching, he worked in a private clinic. He had kindly prepared quite a schedule for me. First he took us out for lunch, which was always a good start. Then he took me to a large community clinic outside town. This was the equivalent to our NHS. Their system is very different from ours and I have described this in the medical part. He and I had a long interview with the medical director which I thought went well. However, she was the only doctor I saw who seemed cross when answering subsequent questions of clarification on emails. I thought about this and decided it may have been that I had not fixed this interview myself, but had just been plonked on her by Mårten, an old colleague.

That evening we were invited to the Kvist household for high tea. It was an unusual treat to be asked home for a meal and it was an entertaining experience. The house was modern in a new development and, like its neighbours, had a sauna (pronounced in Finland, we learnt, 'souna' - the ou as in cow and not mow) upstairs complete with indoor swimming pool. Tea was a family meal with the professor, his new wife Ritta, who is a nurse and works in his clinic, his eighty year old mother-in-law and Ritta's grown-up son and daughter. One of the topics of conversation was the sauna and it became clear that we were expected to join the family in it after tea and probably without any clothes. Now I knew that nothing was going to make me go into this or any other sauna with or without clothes. The thought of some hot steam followed by a cold plunge and being beaten by broomsticks did not appeal to me. I know I must seem like an unadventurous wimp, but having reached the age of seventy and demonstrated with this whole trip that I have not lost the taste for adventure, I decided if there was something I did not want to try I would not.

Anyway, after tea Mårten took me upstairs to his study next to the sauna, where we went on his computer to study academic European medical matters. All the ladies, including Wendy, who you have to admire, went off to the sauna. Ritta sensed Wendy's hesitation and all the ladies including the mother-in-law were provided with swimming costumes. Ritta's son had gone home. After a while the ladies came out and went downstairs. It was getting late now and Mårten closed down his computer and I thought he was going to escort me downstairs so we would go back to our hotel. Instead he went to a cupboard and grabbed a couple of towels but no trunks and started escorting me to the blasted sauna. I just had to dig my heels in and say 'no,' and he did look surprised. I only hope he was not offended. Instead we went into the music room where he gave us a short Chopin piano recital, which to me sounded magical. Then he ran us back to the hotel.

Next morning he took me a short walk to his private clinic where I learnt even more how the Finnish medical system is so different from ours. It is so different that it is impossible to say if it is better but we will come to the factors at the end of the book when I sum up. Afterwards, Wendy and I took him out for lunch and later we took the boat for Stockholm.

Sweden

The ferry to Stockholm was overnight and run by Silja Line. It was the first really good one, big, with spacious, comfortable cabins and two large restaurants, one of which served reindeer meat, which Wendy had for the second time in three days. As we would expect by now, many of the staff were from Eastern Europe and did not speak English. Coming back to the cabin at bedtime after Wendy, I realized I was not sure of my cabin number, which is perhaps not unreasonable after about ten weeks of changing most nights. The key was a blank piece of plastic, which I normally prefer. Every time I asked someone to find out, I was met with a blank stare and eventually had to go down to reception or whatever they call it at sea, and looking rather foolish I was able to get the right information.

When we arrived in the morning, a Friday, we drove straight to Stockholm airport and I dropped Wendy off as she was going home for the weekend to a wedding and to see the family. The plan was for me to stay in Stockholm until Monday, then drive a short way north to Upsalla to see my doctor before moving on to Copenhagen, staying overnight and picking up Wendy on Tuesday. All this went smoothly and I went with Gladys to a boutique hotel on an island in the town centre where I was booked in for three nights. It was an old hotel in the old town with the internet, which the helpful staff could not operate, and no air conditioning.

I enjoyed looking round Stockholm, took some authentic

nonsensical Viking boat trip where there was an amplified guide in all languages which was uninteresting and inaudible. Is it just me or do most city boat trips start out warm and interesting and finish up cold, too long and boring?

One piece of luck was finding the opera house on the second day and it was the first night of *Cavelleria Rusticana* and *I Pagliacci*. For some reason all seats that night were the equivalent of ten euros and I sat in the centre of the second row of the stalls. I spent the whole day in happy anticipation and it was wonderful. Usually I like to go through an opera at home with the CD and the libretto in the weeks before the performance, especially as there would be no English surtitles but I knew these operas quite well and had no difficulty following them.

Talking about surtitles, I think it is a pity more foreign opera houses do not have English surtitles as well as having them in their own language. Certainly in the north of Europe, English must be the most widely spoken language and many people seem fluent in it. It is likely that many in the audience came from outside Sweden and would have followed English surtitles more easily than Swedish. It is possible to have two lots of surtitles simultaneously. As in some towns in Wales for example, the Welsh National Opera have English and Welsh surtitles. I once asked an usher in Llandudno the reason and he told me that he was quite mystified as most of the audience was English and none of the rest spoke Welsh. I know of course that the French would not dream of doing this, but at the Opera Bastille they demonstrate they know the need for it because before the performance starts they have notices on the surtitle screen in French and English about switching off mobile phones. I hope this idea is not seen as chauvinistic arrogance but merely a desire to help people enjoy opera across Europe. I have discovered that at La Scala in Milan surtitles are offered in Italian and English.

I have no idea how they were able to make the seats so cheap yet also available. I love opera but know little about it and cannot say whether it is good or bad. I just know if I like the singing, acting and the sets. I cannot tell any difference in the playing of the orchestra or the conductor.

I usually prefer *Cavelleria Rusticana* and last time I saw it performed, by the Welsh National Opera, I had one of those magical evenings where the singing and the sets excited me so much that I left skipping down the street after; even though that evening I Pagliacci was I thought disappointing with the sets a failure. Well, for this night in Stockholm I did not know what to expect and it turned out to be a revelation. The tenor and soprano had heavenly voices and the set with the church as the centrepiece of the stage worked wonderfully. Better than all of this, though, was the chorus which was large and each voice was to me simply brilliant. After the interval I was expecting the usual anti-climax of I Pagliacci and it was certainly odd seeing it in the same set, a phenomenon I had never come across before. The period chosen was the forties, I believe, and there was a large motorised ice-cream van in front of the church which was used as the home and stage for the strolling players. There was a different cast from Cavelleria Rusticana but it was just as good and the tenor who played Canio, to me, sounded like a world leader. The chorus stayed marvellous and after this double bill I bounded out of the opera house thrilled to the core, the thrill being tempered by the fact that I had no-one to share it with.

These three days of lunches and dinners taken alone were not a success. Mostly I do not find eating on my own a problem, although if the restaurant is busy I wonder if I can detect a reluctance at letting a table for only one. I am quite happy with the newspaper and I was able to get one each day, but the thought of nothing to read is horrific to me. I remember in 1992, we stayed for two nights in Sharrow Bay, where dinner is a long and special event, there were two men on their own at different and adjacent tables. As far as I could see, they did not talk to each other or anyone else except the waiters. Neither had anything to read and they sat there between courses, just looking impassive. I assumed they were enjoying themselves because they must have known what they were doing. It just demonstrates how different folk are.

The best was a Swedish restaurant where a beautiful, slim, almost text-book blonde served me and she was smiling and made me feel at home. The starter, I had learnt not to be adventurous, was based on smoked salmon and gherkin and was fine but the steak was served in a thick sauce which was a mess, literally as well as metaphorically, as this stuff crept up the cutlery on to my fingers. I decided that, as well as having Swedish cooking, I would try a couple of ethnic restaurants. One lunchtime, near the station, I found one of those Chinese buffets where you can eat all you want for a modest amount. There are three of these near where I live and I use them when I want a quick, cheap, pleasant meal. The Stockholm one was similar but not nearly as good.

One evening after having been away too long, I felt my serum curry level was falling again, so I found an Indian restaurant in the old town. It must have been the worst 'Indian' restaurant I have ever been to, even worse then the one I visited in Wick in 1989, with the waiters sullen and very upset to see a customer at nine o' clock. A regular Bangladeshi "Indian" restaurant opening up nearby would have it closed in short order because there must be a level of service the Swedes will not tolerate.

I prefer to eat after theatre performances and this was a problem after the opera. Near the opera house is a narrow, bustling pedestrianised road called DrottningGaten. This was full of pubs and restaurants, most with large outdoor areas, this being August. I left the opera hungry at half past ten, wondering at which of all these places I would choose to eat, when I found to my horror nearly all their kitchens were closed and they were serving drinks only. In the end I found a Spanish bar where, after much grief and pain, they were willing to serve me portions of unpleasant tapas. The unpleasantness was probably because I chose badly, with the head waiter breathing down my neck, implying if I did not choose quickly, there would be no deal.

During some part of each day, I worked on my notes and plans for the next part of the trip. Suddenly I found disaster loomed. According to my notes, the Dutch doctor had not given me an appointment. The plan was for me to ring him for one on the weekend while in Stockholm, before he went on holiday. I phoned and had an automatic message that he was away for two weeks and

I was due to see him a week later. I had found Holland one of the hardest places to arrange a meeting and was frightened that, being holed up in Scandinavia with no contacts, I would be stuck and the whole project would fall apart. Suddenly I remembered that there was a WONCA conference about to start in Florence, because Jean Carl Soler, Gustav Kamenski, Waltraud Fink and Mårten Kvist were all going. I chose Jean Carl Soler, probably because I assumed his first language was English and he was superb. He was just about to go into a meeting but said someone would ring me back and, sure enough, later that morning a Dutch GP called, fully au fait with the problem. Unfortunately he had planned his own holiday when I would be in Holland but he called later with the name and address and contact details of an English-speaking GP in Amsterdam who agreed to see me, and the project was saved.

After I left Stockholm, less than an hour away in Uppsala I had a meeting with a doctor called Karin Lindhagen, a very warm grandmother. We met first at her house, which was full of books, including Shakespeare and other English classics. She took me to lunch at a sort of refectory near the University and then to her surgery for the interview.

Afterwards I planned to drive towards Copenhagen where I had to be at the airport at five o'clock the next day to meet Wendy. I had intended to go about half way and stay at Jonkoping, where I had found a suitable hotel on the Net but I was given so much kind hospitality at Uppsala that by the time I was on my way I realized that I would not get there until about half past nine, which, knowing Sweden, meant there would be no dinner unless I minded being the only guest in a hotel dining room. This happened to Rod and me in Belgrade and, after that and the experience in Bratislava, I decided never again. While driving along a very pleasantly forested road with almost no traffic, I pondered what to do, as you will understand, this is an important problem for me. I vaguely remembered from the map that there was a town about half way to Jonkoping called Linkoping, but I did not know about the hotels, and it is obvious that while being without Google, I was 'non coping'. Anyway, I phoned Lucy who, while sorting out her four daughters, quickly grasped the problem, found the town in a road atlas, searched the internet and gave me the choice of an expensive hotel in the centre of town, which I preferred, or one just off the motorway. She agreed to try and talk the expensive one into a cheap price on the grounds that it was August and not (we thought) a holiday town, and get back to me. Sadly, this hotel was not willing to negotiate so I went to the first, and by joining their point scheme, or whatever, on the spot, got a good deal. Being out of town, I needed a taxi to dinner and, after asking advice from yet another wonderful receptionist, found myself in a Swedish town in an Italian restaurant served by a very civil Portuguese maitre'd.

Denmark

Leaving Sweden, you drive from Malmo straight across the Oresund Bridge into Copenhagen. The bridge is certainly quite some undertaking. It starts as a graceful bridge, then descends onto an island and, a few kilometres later, sinks into a tunnel and as you emerge you are in the outskirts of Copenhagen. I had not realized at the time that under the road bridge was a railway on which trains take about ten minutes to cross between the countries. There were no frontier formalities, just the EU sign saying 'DANMARK', although preceding entry to the bridge you have to pay a massive toll. The airport was on the tunnel side of town, so I picked up Wendy and then drove straight into the city.

Since Danny Kaye and his film *Hans Christian Andersen*, one thinks of 'Wonderful Copenhagen'. Well, it certainly had a lot going for it, but wonderful is probably a bit over the top. In the same way that it is difficult to appreciate good cooking with poor service or a lousy ambience, it is harder to love a place when it is raining. It is even worse when there are problems with the hotel. We were hit with both, so probably I did not give it a fair assessment. Firstly, although it may seem a minor problem to some people, not having a place to park one's car in the immediate vicinity of the hotel, preferably by a valet, is a major inconvenience towards the end of a three month tour. The hotel was not only unable to help with this, but they also provided me with a poorly photocopied map to somewhere that was probably in Germany in order to park the car. I was then expected to walk back.

Secondly, we were given a front bedroom in this fairly upmarket hotel. It looked out onto a busy main road and there was no air-conditioning. As the weather was warm it was impossible to sleep with the windows closed because of the heat and difficult with them open because of the noise. Therefore, if travelling by car or coming in summer, I would advise avoiding the Kong Frederik Hotel.

We stayed in a square near the Tivoli and walked from there to the Amalienborg Palace with the inevitable splendidly uniformed guards and finally to the canal. The architecture was in the Hanseatic style, which we love and which helps to give the place its charm. However, on a beautiful old building in a square someone had perched on the roof an enormous sign just saying 'SAMSUNG'. If some clown working for Samsung wants to get his firm hated he knows how to do it, but you have to see this to believe the Danes would allow such an act of sacrilege. It is probably not right to say it but you do not expect politicians to take bribes in northern parts.

Copenhagen is a city where there are many cyclists and indeed it is encouraged by the authorities in a most charming way. We came across a cycle park where the bikes all had their own characteristic shape and colour. They were locked by supermarket trolley style chains, and one merely had to deposit a coin to release the chain and ride away. I mean deposit, not fee, because the money comes out when the chain is put back. On the front of the cycle a hard map is fixed showing the city and outlining the area in which you are permitted to take it.

We arrived in Copenhagen on a Tuesday and the next morning I had a twenty minute walk to see my doctor, Bodil Johnsen, who had a Danish snack waiting for me. Wendy as usual was able to find a guided tour of some aspect of the town and this is what she did this morning. In fact, in Copenhagen she was the only customer so had a very private tour. Incidentally, when my visit includes lunch, Wendy has to find her own alone and she also likes to read then.

Holland

For the first time since Budapest we had to drive so far between capitals that we had to stop overnight. We stayed in Bremen, back in Germany, on the way to Holland where, as in all the small countries, we saw only the capital. Amsterdam has some of the characteristics of Copenhagen, but they are all exaggerated. Although the latter is thought to be a cycling city, it is nothing compared with the former. They are everywhere; indeed, cycling seems to be the main form of transport in the city. The GP I called on does her visits by bicycle, and in fact it is the only way she could get around. It would not be correct to say the cycle is king-of-the-road; it vies for this position with the pedestrian. Motorists are the serfs and the roads are organised to make them know their place. We found our hotel, the Krasnapolsky, on the other side of Dam Square and after two circles trying to get to it with the satellite navigation we gave up. Wendy got in a taxi and I followed. The driver did half the circle and then seemed to go down roads away from the hotel for about twenty minutes at a snail's pace. During this time I was sweating blood because although we had started with plenty of time I was now getting late for my appointment. This was on a Friday afternoon and not only was the doctor waiting for me but it will be remembered that this was the appointment arranged at short notice for me via Florence through a Maltese and a Dutch doctor while I was in Stockholm. It was a relief when suddenly the hotel appeared before us like an oasis.

The Krasnapolsky is a luxury hotel we had yearned to stay in since hearing it praised by Wendy's parents over thirty years ago, when we could only dream of such opulence. It was as great as expected but was marred, only slightly, by the need to pay for use of the internet on my laptop. With this pettiness, a hotel could never be perfect.

We checked in and then I took another taxi to see Dr Joke Schulkes-van de Pol, a very glamorous lady looking much younger than her age. This consultation had an extra interest because Dutch general practice had always worked closely with British general practice and, ever since I can remember, there have been articles written by Dutch GPs in the British Medical Journal. Our practice used the Dutch guidelines to treat ear infections of children. (I come to the use of guidelines in *The Medical Part*.) Joke was too busy to meet us in the evening but she recommended a Chinese restaurant near the hotel, which was enormous, and we went there that night. It was on a pedestrian road, very noisy and dirty and teeming with tourists. The room was large but the waitres, from Hong Kong, was friendly.

As I had had my appointment on Friday, the next day was a holiday and we spent it just walking along the canals in the old town. The city is also built with wonderful Hanseatic style buildings but Dam Square and the roads immediately off it are brash and overcrowded. It takes only a few minutes to get away from there and the city becomes an area of quiet canals with narrow pavements and all sorts of curious shops. The peaceful feeling of being along these roads is an efficacious antidote to the frenetic buzz of the centre.

We bought things from stalls, at least Wendy did, but mainly we strolled. It was a cloudy day, but quiet where we were and we loved it. We found the road with the Indonesian restaurants and booked a meal for the evening. We always have a rijsttafel, which means 'rice table', while in Amsterdam. It is a mixture of many European and Far Eastern cuisines that originally came from the Dutch East Indies. I cannot describe it here but you just order one course and a whole load of small dishes come, many of rice and of varying degrees of spiciness.

107

One thing we noticed in Europe was that pedestrians waited for green crossing lights. In many countries, people seem to wait until the lights change, sometimes when there is no traffic in sight. Well, Amsterdam is not like that in the centre. When people want to cross a road they just cross, doing a waltz round the cycles. Cars are just ignored and have no other option but crawling along and frequently stopping.

There is another point about being out on the roads in Europe, and that is I had the impression that the sirens or bells of emergency vehicles are not heard with anything like the frequency that you come across them in England. This could of course be a false impression but I wonder if there are statistics available.

Belgium

We arrived in Brussels after an easy drive on a Sunday morning and Gladys guided us straight to our hotel. In the afternoon Sylvia and Edgar arrived and I was excited as I had not seen them since they joined us in Italy. We took a bus to the Grand' Place, probably the most splendid square we saw, but I may be forgetting Rome, Salamanca and Madrid. I cannot understand why Brussels is not at first thought a major centre of tourism. People flock to Paris, Prague and Tallinn; many can picture the canals in Amsterdam or the Danube in Budapest but to many, Brussels is a closed book. The Grand Place is in the centre of the old town, which can only be described as stunning. Facing each other in this square must be a couple of the most breath-taking buildings in Europe. However, that is not all, for surrounding the place are a myriad of old, narrow, beautiful streets which are lovely to walk along.

When we arrived, there was a beer festival in progress and it was so crowded that you had to go to a booth on the perimeter to buy vouchers for the beer. They are proud of the enormous number of varieties of Belgian beer there are and it appeared that the total is about the same as the population, if you bear in mind Belgium is a small country. A bus ride away from the Place is the European Parliament, but that is another story.

The receptionist in our hotel, a Marriott, was in a sunny mood and gave us upgrades to club class rooms. This entitled us to use the club lounge, which provided free food and drink in the early evenings. The hospitality was warm but I could not see the point of it. Each sandwich I ate, and they were good, made me guilty that I would lose my appetite for dinner and once I start these things, if they are that good I find it hard to stop. That night we went to a restaurant we had booked by The Grand' Place but it was not marvelous, spoilt by a surly waiter who I believe was Belgian and not Polish. On our second night in Brussels we ate nearer the hotel and this was a good recommendation from the concierge.

On the Monday I had my interview with my Belgian doctor. I recruited him by means of his neighbour, who is English and also his patient. This neighbour is a friend of Rod's who contacted him and arranged the email introduction. Dr Hariga picked me up and returned me to the hotel. The meeting with him had an added interest because not only was he single-handed but he had no practice staff at all. Although I was to come across this phenomenon to a certain extent in Luxembourg and France, it was the first time I had seen it and I was, and still am, amazed. We will look at staff in *The Medical Part*.

Luxembourg

Luxembourg is, as is well known, the smallest of the twenty five EU members (in 2006) and the capital has the same name. Although small, it is certainly independent in its approach to general practice. I met two GPs together in the offices of their academic college of general practice. They were ferociously proud of their freedoms to the extent that they will not even allow their government to force them to keep up to date. More on these doctors will come to light in *The Medical Part*.

I talked to them about Europe. They are passionately in favour of the EU and, although I accept this was a small and unrepresentative group, I thought this could be how most people felt. I think it is something to do with being such a small country; they feel happier being part of a large federation.

As a digression, it saddens me that in the UK, if not everywhere, views are polarized about the EU. There are those who are pleased with it, see the benefits and would like it to continue as it is, warts and all. The opposing party, as well as valuing our old traditions, object to being ruled by bureaucrats in Brussels, want to keep the pound and wish Britain had never joined. I find it difficult to meet anyone with my view in Europe or at home that the EU is a wonderful organization, should become wider and deeper; but we should not be ruled by those bureaucrats in Brussels but by a properly elected federal parliament, using a system of government similar to the United States. And like the United States, if the president has any power, he should be elected by the people. Thus we could be proud Europeans without being alienated.

Unfortunately, our hotel was at the edge of town by the airport. It was a Sheraton, but rather than posh was more of a budget range hotel. In spite of these factors, surprisingly it turned out to be one of the nicest we found on the whole tour. This was due to the attitude of the staff, especially the receptionists. As well as being well informed and helpful, they always seemed delighted to talk to us, greeted us by name and generally gave us a feel-good factor. When we left, I sought out the assistant manager on duty and told him what I thought.

The city was too difficult to understand in the short time I was there. It seemed to have an upper town and a lower one. I was in only the upper part but when walking across bridges over the gorges, I could look down onto the countryside so far below. I had no clue how to get down there and as far as I could see there were no lifts. The view, though, made me think it would be worthwhile to make the descent one day. Unfortunately, I did not have time to sort it out. The roads going into the centre were wide and one had a feeling of ease and pleasure driving along them but I suspect that this may be different in rush hour. In the hours I spent with the doctors, including lunch, Wendy went on a guided walking tour of both the upper and lower towns and came back with her eyes shining, insisting we return for a weekend the following year.

France

France has always been my favourite country after the UK, probably because it is so different from us that it makes the thought of going abroad such an adventure. The motorways work well, mostly with little traffic.

I have little to say about France or Paris that you do not already know. If you have not been to these places, you have lost out and I advise you to look for your diaries, oil your credit cards and get to both as soon as possible. However, keep them out of sight in Paris and on the south coast. The cliché about the restaurants and cooking having excellent food in general is, in my experience, as true as ever. However, obviously, clichés about the French being rude and charming cannot both be true and I have usually found they are the latter. Even the few who lack the charisma to give you the 'feel-good factor' are invariably polite.

On the Thursday afternoon we drove from Luxembourg to Paris for our last capital and country. The doctor was an English doctor called Sarah Hartley, who lived with her husband and children. She had been a GP and now specialized in sleep medicine. However, she was my contact and she had made arrangements for me to see a GP the next day.

As mentioned in the section on Austria, I have always had a horror of staying in other people's homes. I am comfortable with the routine in mine, and happy arranging a routine in hotels. I am not sure what makes me turn down invitations to stay with friends in their homes or holiday cottages. It may be loss of control but it is more a feeling that I don't want to seem fussy with my own routines. We sleep with two pillows each and have done so for so long that less than this would cause terminal insomnia. Wendy looks for these on being shown to a hotel room and if not there, asks for them. As a guest of a friend, I am not sure that this is the right thing to do. I feel that one should be grateful for what one gets on the analogy if you accept a dinner invitation you must eat and pretend to enjoy what you are given, even if it is a dish that revolts you.

Even more important than this are the lavatory arrangements. We have a bathroom-en-suite at home so there is no embarrassment for us when we have guests, and wherever we stay in hotels and the like, our bedroom has private facilities, even when on a rice boat in South India. I have a horror amounting almost to a phobia of sitting on a loo when someone in the household tries the door. Indeed, strangely, I have always felt embarrassed that anybody should even know that I am I there. I suppose you would call this a sort of neurotic introversion, which Freud might have understood.

Anyway, three doctors invited us to stay with them and in two cases it was impossible to refuse without jeopardizing the project. I was terrified for days in advance. In the first case, as we saw in Austria, our hostess was a middle-aged single lady living in a large house. Paris was the second experience of this and what made it worse was that it was for two nights. This was in a small chateau on three floors with a family who had four bright children, in fact two pairs of twins. Our bedroom was on the first floor and although large with a balcony overlooking green rolling hills there was no bath or lavatory off it. Opposite was the master bedroom, which Wendy had discovered had it own private facilities. Next to our room was a lavatory without a lock, and therefore no use to me at all, and, opposite, a large bathroom which included a mirror and a toilet and a lock. Wendy discovered that the children slept on the second floor and had their own toilet facilities. All would have been well except that on the shelf over the basin were four brightly coloured electric tooth brushes each in its distinctive mug, staring at me like a firing squad. Fortunately, I was able to manage by waiting until all the children went to bed.

It is a pity about all this neurotic nonsense of mine, which I must point out Wendy does not share, because our two stays in homes turned out to be the high points of the holiday.

The house was in a suburb called St Cloud, Cloud being pronounced 'cloo'. There was no regular address and Gladys had to rely on the postcode, but this was hopeless, as French post codes cover a much larger area than the UK. Eventually we found the village and a kind man, who had been a patient of Sarah's, did the only possible thing and got in the car and directed us round the windy, narrow one-way streets of St Cloud to Sarah's home. Fortunately, we had almost completed a circle so our friend had only a short downhill walk back to where we met him. This house itself was fascinating, for as well as being built on three floors, it had a tower, complete with battlements on top.

The family was very welcoming and we had a lovely dinner of beef fillet, followed by cheese, with Sarah and her husband Julian, who is a financial adviser.

The next day, Sarah, after some trouble with her car causing her to be too late to put me on the train for my appointment, drove me to the office in Paris where I was to meet my doctor and then went on with Wendy to have coffee and a croissant in the centre before going on to her work. Wendy enjoyed herself walking round the Parisian shops before finishing up at the Musée d'Orsay.

My doctor was Jean Brami, who is a professor of general practice in the University of Paris. We met in an office where he helps to organize and modernize French general practice. Afterwards, he took me by metro to lunch on the Rue de Rivoli and then showed me his surgery nearby. When we had finished, I walked to the Musée d'Orsay and rejoined Wendy for more walking.

In the evening we took Sarah and Julian to a local bistro, which to us was more like a good restaurant with a splendid menu; I can still remember the kidneys. There was of course the usual problem of the wine list. As always in France, it was vast and divided into regions and had names of châteaux which meant nothing to me. The years varied but I don't carry a table of which year is good in each region and the only other thing I could understand was the price, which varied from many hundreds of euros to an affordable figure. I often wonder how many punters could tell the difference between a thousand euro bottle of wine and a two thousand euro bottle from the same area in a double blind trial. Except for the odd connoisseur who might just happen to be dining in a bistro in St Cloud, the whole thing seems to be a bit of a nonsense to me. In the end, I solved the problem by asking Julian which wine he normally drank here and ordered that. However, this is still no guidance in choosing wine when in France.

Another issue in French restaurants is the comparison of the way they serve cheese compared with England. I like the way it is usually part of a set meal and the presentation on trolleys so that you can choose small portions from a wide variety of cheeses. I know it is unsophisticated, but I miss Cheddar and Stilton, although Roquefort if nice and creamy, makes up for it. I can never understand the way it is usually served in England. It is usually a separate or additional course, more expensive than the other desserts, less choice and, worst of all, comes in much too large portions. As a consequence, I rarely order it in London. Perhaps I should start a national restaurant cheese boycott until restaurateurs take the point and serve a wider and cheaper choice of smaller portions.

Lastly on cheese, but not restaurants, is whether it should be served before the dessert, as in France, or after as in England. I am not really bothered about this but cheese is moreish and it is nice to go on nibbling at it over coffee and port or a liqueur.

Really finally about restaurants is the old problem of tipping. I have learnt that you are either for it or against it and can no more convince anyone who disagrees than you can about religious belief, political allegiance or even whether the death penalty should be restored. However, you will realize by now that I cannot resist stating my case. This is that waiting staff do a job and they should be paid the right rate and as a customer I should be charged the correct amount to cover the restaurateur's costs and profit and that is it. If the wages are unfairly small, it is not my problem, as I consider it the management's task to work out pay and prices. If they can do it for the chefs and cleaners, they can do it for waiters. I find tipping patronizing and embarrassing. It is of course worse with chip and pin, when I am handed a machine and have to do some sort of maths while half cut after a large amount of food and drink. I have taken to telling the waiter to add the usual tip himself. I have no interest in rewarding good service or penalizing bad. I expect it to be good anyway and that is a factor in my choice of restaurants. If it is bad I will not return and occasionally may make a complaint. Americans tell me that if the food takes too long to come they may reduce the tip, but that ignores the fact that the problem could be in the kitchen.

Conclusions

Was it worth it? The answer is in no doubt for me and it is 'Yes' without any hesitation. The major problems were fixing the doctors' appointments, but everything else was routine. I suppose organizing the drive to Cyprus could also be called difficult but nothing else. Fixing the ferries was hard work, which needed persistence, but was not really a problem. I did not have time to book the hotels myself and this I regret because it would have been something I would have enjoyed, but with all my criteria Wexas did not do too badly.

It is not too much of an oversimplification to say that, apart from meeting the doctors, this was like any other motoring holiday only longer. As we have seen, there were problems with frontiers in Eastern Europe but the only ones that mattered were the ones anywhere around Turkey. The new EU countries have not really got the idea how to run their borders now they are in the Union and these arbitrary choices of looking at Green Cards or Car Registration Documents implies that they never knew what they were doing anyway. I would advise any driver motoring in those areas to make sure that they take both.

We knew we were lucky in that nothing went wrong in the four major risk areas, namely our health, the health of the car, accidents and bandits. What the risks were in percentage terms, I never discovered. Obviously we were as careful as possible.

This was a great motoring holiday for people like us who enjoy this sort of thing, the driving of a nice car, seeing new countries, sleeping in some great hotels and of course always looking forward to a special dinner each night. For me, it never became repetitious, even being away for so long; perhaps this was because of the excitement of interviewing the doctors. There were of course disadvantages, including not seeing my family for so long and having only a superficial look at the countries and towns we went through, but of course we can and will return to those we found interesting. Lastly, although we had been married for forty four years, I found I got to know Wendy better, and after forty seven years I knew much more about Rod.

THE MEDICAL PART
The Doctors

As you would expect, the doctors were a very mixed bunch. However, the ones that had agreed to be interviewed by me were usually friendly. Most were ordinary GPs but a few were academics and some were medical teachers, training future family doctors.

The usual procedure was for me to have an appointment, I would find my way to their surgery and after a two to three hour interview would return to my hotel.

However many doctors did more than the minimum. Often they picked me up and returned me to my hotel and sometimes they took me out to lunch, or Wendy and I to dinner. On these occasions, as we have seen, we had a much better meal than we could have found ourselves.

All spoke English well enough for the interview but some seemed to be at least bilingual. Surprisingly, many had never been to the UK or even lived in an English-speaking area, having learnt their English only at school. None spoke English with an American accent.

I have impressed on all of them that they must contact me if ever they come to Britain because I would love to see them again and show them round. There have been some exchanges of Christmas cards.

Although about half the doctors I saw were male, I had the impression that there were more female doctors in many countries.

In Cyprus, for example, the doctor I saw did her shift from 7.30 in the morning until 2.30 in the afternoon, and these hours of course fit in well for mothers meeting their children from school. As far as I could make out, doctors on the continent did not do both morning and evening surgeries, unlike in the UK. In many countries, the day's work finished in the mid afternoon and in others the doctor did one long surgery a day and varied the times. For example, the one that I saw in Budapest worked from eight o'clock in the morning until noon on some days and from three in the afternoon until seven o'clock in the evenings on others.

The system of pay, as we shall see in the next chapter, varies enormously from country to country, but in those countries where the doctors are paid each time they see the patient, the GPs tend to be single-handed and more flexible, and will see patients whenever it is mutually convenient. Although this might seem to have many advantages, it cannot work in the UK, where practices are large and doctors work with a team of ancillary staff, which would be difficult to assemble for one-off consultations.

Money Matters

Money is obviously an important feature of all countries. We must consider it from the point of view of patients and doctors. Also we need to consider the mechanism that each country uses to transfer money from the former to the latter.

Let us get the system out of the way first. Basically patients pay money to 'a system' and this system pays the doctors. I am sure no one imagines that health care is free. In the UK patients pay the government in National Insurance and taxes and then the government pays the doctors. Other countries have different systems. Some use the local community, which is equivalent to an English borough council, others insurance societies, and in Greece the trade unions are responsible. As far as we are concerned, the actual system used in any particular country is not important so I use terms like the national health, the authorities or the system interchangeably. Even in countries like Ireland, where patients see GPs privately; there will be exempt groups such as the long term unemployed, so there will be a 'system' in place for arranging their treatment with the doctors.

Ireland is the only country where general practice is totally private. The doctor charges a fee for every consultation. Dr Shearer, whose practice I visited, told me that he charges forty-five euros for the first consultation of any illness and thirty for subsequent ones. The fee for house calls is higher. This may seem a lot, but it is his only income and he has to pay all his practice expenses out of this.

In Malta, the general practice is almost private, in that about eighty percent of GPs there are private, although they look after about sixty six percent of the patients. The consultation charge there is between seven and ten euros. This seems very cheap compared with Ireland, but the state doctors are paid in the region of twenty two thousand euros a year, so perhaps the cost of living is low there. In those countries where patients have to pay up front, either privately or with a rebate, they will be charged more for a house call.

In some other countries, the patients have to pay, but only a little, towards their treatment, the rest coming from the state. For example, in Portugal the patients pay a nominal fee of two euros each time, although there are many exemptions. In some countries, France, Luxembourg and Belgium for example, the patient pays for all his treatment but gets a substantial rebate from the state. The French social security system is quite complicated in that doctors are placed on one of three lists, the first list charging the lowest and the rates rising through list two, reaching a maximum in list three. There are very few GPs on list three, less than one per cent, and most GPs in large cities are on list two. Patients get the same amount of money reimbursed whether they see doctors on the first or second list, which when I was there was seventy percent of twenty one euros. The rebate for attending list three doctors is very small. This, to a certain extent, is similar in Belgium where many doctors work in a government health insurance scheme, where the fees are agreed. Some doctors work outside this system and they can charge what they like, but patients get a smaller proportion of rebate, as the amount repaid is fixed even though the doctor may have charged more.

In Finland, which in so many respects is different from anywhere else, patients have to pay as well. In the community practice that I visited they paid either a subscription of twenty two euros, which covers them for a year, or eleven euros for each consultation. On top of this they must pay fifteen euros for any failure to attend appointments and fifteen euros for any out-of hours visit.

Now let us look at the doctors' pay. They can be paid a salary, capitation fees or by a mixture of capitation fees and items of service payments. When doctors are paid a salary, for example in Cyprus, Portugal and Sweden, this is often the whole of their state income. Capitation fees are a sum paid by the state to a GP for every patient on his list or registered with his practice. The main way general practitioners are paid in the UK is by capitation fee, with nothing extra for house calls. The rate varies a bit but is in the region of fifty four pounds per patient per year. However, in the UK GPs are also paid a lot extra for achieving various targets under the Quality and Outcomes framework (QOF). These targets are mostly concerned with treating illness to a high standard, often using guidelines laid down by the state. Doctors must keep lists of patients suffering from many conditions and then must treat them in a certain way and help the patient to gain a required outcome. For example, when treating high blood pressure in diabetics the doctor must, amongst the drugs he uses, choose a preparation from one of two groups, unless there are medical reasons why this choice would be unsuitable. He must also demonstrate that he has reduced the blood pressure to 145/85 or less. In addition there are also targets for practice organization, including some provision for the practice to make it reasonably easy (at least in theory) to get an appointment. These extra payments are considerable and are awarded on a point system. A large practice can earn about one thousand points a year and is paid two hundred and fifty pounds per point.

Germany uses an unusual variation of the capitation fee system. The doctors are paid seventy euros each quarter for each patient on their list, and the patient has to pay ten euros once each quarter and then all the rest of the GP's services are free. However, for the doctor, there is a rub in that if the patient does not return after three months, the contract is ended and he gets no further pay until the patient re-attends. Contrast this with the British arrangements in which the doctor is paid the capitation fee regardless of when, if ever, the patient uses his services.

In some countries the only payment doctors get is being paid for what they actually do and this method is known as 'items of service'. This means the doctors are paid for every consultation in the surgery and also for house calls, these usually being at a higher rate.

125

This system can be in the private sector, as in Ireland, but is also used in state systems such as Belgium and Luxembourg. Usually in these systems the patients pay up front and a proportion is reimbursed by the state.

Some countries have a mixed capitation fee and item of service system. In Denmark, for example, the capitation fee accounts for thirty percent of a doctor's pay and the rest is for items of service. In Holland, the trend is reversed and here capitation fees are about sixty percent of the income with a supplement for people aged sixty five and over and for urban deprived areas. The other forty percent is an item of service payment. There is a fixed fee of nine Euros for every face to face consultation and a bigger fee of thirteen and a half euros for home visits. There is a smaller fee of four and a half euros for telephone consultations and the same for an email consultation. If a face to face consultation goes on longer than twenty minutes the doctor is allowed to charge for a double consultation. The doctors have assistants who also give consultations and can charge for them. Holland is the only country where I was told the GPs were paid for telephone and email consultations.

As in Holland, in all cases where the doctors get fees for items of service, either from patients or the state, these are increased for home visits. The rates vary and, where small, do not encourage house calls as they are not considered cost-effective. In Austria, however, when we come to look at house visits, we will see that they are well paid for these and are therefore happy to do them.

I was told, off the record, that in one country the method of payment had been capitation fees only but the state wanted to encourage the doctors to do more for their patients and to be more available so the system was changed to a mixed one. A doctor elsewhere told me that in his country, although technically illegal, doctors tend to accept an envelope with cash in from patients when they make house calls and this seems to be accepted on both sides. Also, some patients hand envelopes of cash to the doctors after a face to face consultation at surgery. These sums appear to be quite small, seemingly in the range of about two to three euros.

Whatever system is used, there can be enhancements, which are often small. For example, the doctor I met in Hungary told me he was paid at a rate increased by a factor of 1.2 times the usual rate for his services as he had been a specialist in internal medicine before he entered general practice. In some countries, as used to be the case in the UK, the doctor is paid more for older patients on his list. In Spain there is a small reward for generic prescribing and this is a subject we will return to later. At present, Dutch GPs are paid an extra fee if their practices participate in a diabetic protocol. This is apparently not a big thing such as the QOF payments earned by our doctors mentioned above.

Types of Practice

As in the UK, general practices come in a variety of sizes, from single doctors to large groups. At each end of the range, however, there are extremes.

Being an independent doctor is quite common in Europe, both east and west, but strangely it is possible to be extremely single-handed where the doctor is not only on his own but, as I saw in Belgium and other places, has no staff at all. We will see more about this when we review staff later.

Many doctors became single-handed in Eastern Europe from about 1991 as a result of Perestroika. Before that time they worked as employees in big polyclinics run by the state and were both salaried and very heavily managed. Lately their governments have encouraged them to go 'private'. This does not mean private practice but that doctors provide their own premises and run a National Health-type practice as a business, similar to us in the UK. They value their new found freedom and this does have implications in that I found some to have no interest in guidelines or audits. This made it quite clear that they no longer wanted any interference. If they are not alone, they work in small groups.

There are paradoxes to the single-handed state. For example, the doctor I saw in Slovakia worked in a building which included a whole range of specialists as well as the GPs. There was a total of forty doctors practising there. It was quite clear, though, that the GPs were firmly independent and that, apart from covering each other for holidays, they had little to do with each other. Unlike group practice, if a doctor had a difficult clinical problem and wanted advice, he would not call in one of his colleagues from the health centre. However, in Portugal, where the doctors do work in groups, I had the impression that they were lonely and did not interact with each other.

Group practice was fairly common and practices of three doctors was probably the most frequent figure I came across. Some of these appeared to be partnerships but those that I went to in Italy and Slovenia were owned by one or more of the doctors and in the latter case, one of the owners was a specialist. The status of the employed GPs in the Italian practice was not clear but their income and workload was less than the owner. This was because the owner had been there the longest, was better known and therefore had more patients, and this determined the proportion of income. The non-owning GPs in the Slovenian practice were salaried employees.

When doctors in Cyprus work in small groups, the doctors are appointed by the state and the partners have no say in this. Some countries, such as Finland and Sweden, provide group practice owned and run by the local community and the doctors are salaried.

At the other extreme were the big groups. In Finland, Portugal (where the practice I visited had forty-one doctors and fifteen nurses), Spain (fourteen GPs) and Malta, doctors work in large groups, even larger than the UK, and there is little continuity of care. In Finland, the health centre had seventeen GPs and five trainees and patients may be assigned to any doctor for their appointment. Although these were all GPs, actual or in training, there was some specialisation amongst them. For example, two did most of the difficult diabetes and very little else. The straightforward Type ll diabetics were looked after by all the doctors. Another two looked after the primary care beds in the clinic and also any visits and, again, this took up most of their time.

The size of the practice has some influence on continuity of care. Obviously this should be good in the independent practices, however in some countries, such as Belgium and Luxembourg, patients are free to visit any GP at any time and get the same reimbursement. In Belgium, however, I was told that the insurance agency had kept figures and noticed that eighty percent of patients kept to the same doctor.

Continuity of care was harder to assess in the small groups. It seems that there is variation of continuity of care in these practices and this variation is probably similar to the UK. In Sweden there was a nice compromise in that the staff divides the patients into two groups, one prefers their own doctor and see their own doctor when available; while the other group do not mind which doctor they see and the nurses have no difficulty fitting them in anywhere.

Finland has other problems with continuity of care, apart from the size of their community health clinics. These problems are caused by there being three primary care systems. As well as the community health centre where they are registered, there are private GPs, and also there is an occupational health service. In Finland some patients get free prescriptions while others have part of the cost reimbursed by the authorities. Patients seeing a private GP have the same rebates for their medicines as they do when they attend the community clinic. I was given the impression that more people attended the private clinics, at least some of the time, than in the UK. There are various reasons for this, including wanting a personal doctor, the proximity of the private clinic to their work and, of course, the prescription payment rebate. The occupational health service is provided by employers, who must have a contract with an occupational health physician and the minimum would be to determine that it is safe for the patient to do the job. Many employers pay a higher fee to the occupational doctor in order to provide a full range of GP services. They may work in community centres or private clinics, depending on the level of contract they have with the employers. Again these doctors prescribe for their patients, even for chronic disease, who are able to obtain their medication on the same terms as the state system. There is no sharing of records between the community GPs, the private doctors and the occupational health physicians.

In other countries, Malta being an example, the private and state primary systems run side-by-side, each being able to allow patients the same range of subsidised prescriptions, in competition and not communicating with each other.

The range of practices I saw throughout Europe closely mirrors the UK, although I had the impression that there was less variation within each country. There was a large range of size of surgery. In Belgium and Austria, where I visited two doctors in different parts of the state, the doctors were single-handed but also practiced from home, although one of the Austrian GPs had moved out to a larger house in the village. Some surgeries were in shops, others in office blocks and others were purpose-built and large.

In Tallinn, the practice was a group of four up a couple of floors in a polyclinic built in the thirties under a different regime. They were slightly unusual in that I entered a large waiting room with many doors leading off it, all labelled in Estonian. There were no staff in sight to report to and I had to find an English-speaking patient to tell me which door to open to find the receptionist.

Surgeries in office blocks were sometimes obscure, with no indication outside that doctors practised there. I had to trust I had the right address and go through the front door to find either a notice or a concierge to direct me. In many European countries most graduates have the title doctor so it was interesting to see that the signs said "Dr med B…"

Some countries had fine, modern, purpose-built health centres. These included Spain and Cyprus but the most remarkable was the community health centre just outside Turku in Finland. It is a polyclinic with other specialities and serves the whole of its community and a smaller neighbouring one. It is responsible for twenty nine thousand inhabitants. In the clinic are wards with a total of eighty beds, which the doctors told me proudly were primary care beds. The clinic is modern, built in the 1980s and 1990s, and very spacious. In the waiting room at the reception desk, patients sit down to speak to the receptionist and there is a green line on the floor behind which waiting patients must stand so that they do not overhear the conversation. I thought this was a very nice touch, as in the UK the patient waiting to speak to the receptionist is often able to overhear the conversation of his predecessor. Also in Britain, the receptionist usually doubles up as the telephonist and the patient at the counter can hear the whole phone conversation where there is a risk of serious breaches of confidentiality. At the clinic in Finland, there is also a small café in the waiting room.

In Europe many doctors work in polyclinics where there are plenty of specialities on site, including primary healthcare paediatricians and primary healthcare gynaecologists (see *Range of work*). Polyclinics were a feature of Eastern Europe before Perestroika and remain in some places, such as Slovakia and Estonia, but in other countries such as the Czech Republic and Poland there is a move to break away from these and the doctors welcome the freedom of independent practice with little supervision.

All the consulting suites that I saw were well-equipped sometimes superbly so. Being single-handed did not seem to have an adverse effect on this. In Austria, for example, both surgeries I saw had a physiotherapy room although the physiotherapist in one of them was on maternity leave and there was no locum. One of the Austrian surgeries had an auto analyser, operated mainly by the HCA equivalents. (HCA stands for Health Care Assistants, a comparatively modern type of nurse replacement in the UK, which we will come to later when we discuss practice staff.) I seem to have seen ECG equipment in every surgery I visited.

There is a body is called PHARE which is a European organisation whose function is to help the accession states which joined the EU in 2004 in a variety of ways. Some help was given to GPs in Lithuania, when they were encouraged to move into privately-owned surgeries and they were helped to buy some pathology equipment. This help has now stopped except in Eastern Lithuania, which is significantly poorer than Vilnius.

Range of Work

The British way of general practice is for the doctor to be responsible for all illnesses from the cradle to the grave for the patients registered on his list. This concept has a great bearing on the way we keep our records, and from there, how we manage to treat many common diseases. We will explore these subjects later. However, to my amazement, this is not the case in many European countries. The main exceptions are looking after children (paediatrics) and women's complaints (gynaecology).

In the UK and many countries on the continent, paediatricians and gynaecologists are usually hospital specialists. For example, the former, among other responsibilities, will manage premature babies in incubators, while the latter are experienced in major surgery such as operating on cancer of the womb or doing caesarean sections. What I discovered was that in some places there are specialists trained only to work in primary care, to whom the patients go direct. These therefore act as GPs for children and ladies with women's complaints. I must repeat our system requires that these patients come to us first, where we are trained to treat children and women, and to see specialists only if we refer them.

Let us look at primary care paediatricians first. Some of these work in polyclinics, but others are on their own. The age of change over from paediatrician to GP varies between the countries. In Hungary, for example, the patient or parents can choose and from the age of seven to eighteen they can decide whether to continue to attend a paediatricians rather than their GP.

In some countries, although it may be common for GPs to look after children, others feel a loss of confidence in this field and will not register them until they have reached a given age. There is always the alternative of the primary care paediatrician with no extra cost to the patient. As I have stressed, this option is not available for British GPs and their child patients, but District General Hospitals (DGHs) usually have specialists on duty who would see a child for a GP when asked.

In Austria, the GPs do look after children from birth but, having no nurses, do all the immunisation injections themselves. They are also required to do regular health checks on babies; for example, the doctor I interviewed told me that he will do four checks personally in the first year, including doing measurements such as height, weight and head circumference. He told me that he has never picked up any severe illnesses while doing these examinations but has found several minor conditions. Until about 1990 GPs in the UK did these examinations, although not so many. However, because we hardly ever discovered anything wrong that the mothers had not already brought to our attention we found these so called 'well baby clinics' a poor use of time. These check-ups in the UK ever since have mostly been done by health visitors, but the number of check ups has been reduced.

In Britain, baby immunisations are usually given by nurses or health visitors but in the rest of the EU, with few exceptions, they are given by doctors, either GPs or paediatricians. It is said that great perturbation would result if these were done by a nurse. I heard this early on in Greece, which was the fifth country I had come to, but it was repeated often afterwards. GPs, even when they did their own paediatrics, knew of no targets for immunisations, but most countries seem to achieve high levels by having a requirement that it must be demonstrated that the immunisation programme is up to date before a child can start school.

In many countries the position with regard to primary care gynaecology is similar. Their main role is to be available for patients with gynaecological symptoms but they also do cervical smears (which are usually done by GPs' nurses here), ultrasounds, including, where necessary, through the vagina, checking bone density for thinning of bones (osteoporosis), and monitoring pregnancy by ultrasound scans and blood tests. Some patients are likely to turn to them first with breast problems.

There is enormous variation about this. In Slovenia I was told that it is illegal for GPs to do vaginal examinations. In other countries, although not illegal, it would be unthinkable. GPs in many other countries could do gynaecology if they wanted but usually left it to the primary care gynaecologists. In these places they thought that younger GPs who had done some gynaecology during their training for general practice might still be willing to carry on doing it themselves. Paradoxically I learnt that in Belgium it is the younger doctors who prefer to avoid gynaecology and that patients usually go straight to primary care gynaecologists. This is more expensive, with a smaller rebate than if they go to clinics, and many go to private gynaecologists where there may be no rebate. The smaller rebate matters in poorer areas where patients would not want to spend this extra money and would still expect their GPs to do gynaecology. Of course, in these countries the women's' choice would be important.

This practice in many countries, where paediatrics and gynaecology are done not by GPs but by primary care paediatricians or gynaecological specialists, is an important notion for English GPs to grasp, especially in London and other urban areas where many European patients are living. Often foreign ladies have come to me and have started a consultation by saying that their baby needs a referral to a paediatrician or they need a referral to a gynaecologist and seemed disconcerted when I asked them why. An appreciation of the different systems of other countries would have saved me much mutual misunderstanding.

General practice is still fairly new in Greece and, although being developed, is not widely available. Primary care is usually available in large health centres staffed entirely by specialists, including internists (physicians), who will do much of what would be general practice in other countries. There are also primary care paediatricians, primary care gynaecologists, dentists and pathologists. In the countryside, there are small satellite clinics in villages, looking after only a few hundred patients. When doctors qualify in Greece, they have to do a compulsory year's military service, where they may learn some more medicine; on leaving the army they then have to work by law for a year staffing these satellite centres. During this year, they have no supervision and no further training or education, but can refer difficult cases to the health centre. This equivalent of general practice by a doctor in training working in such an isolated way, would not be allowed in the UK.

Access

Access is a term used to mean how easy it is for patients to make contact with their doctor. This, apart from arranging consultations, also means how easy is it to get to speak to him on the phone or even, as is now coming in, having an email consultation. Lastly it means how possible is it to arrange a home visit.

As we make comparisons with the rest of Europe, we will look at the position here, and the best way to put it is that it is patchy. Most British doctors work by appointment and the delay to get one was, until about a few years ago, much more variable than doctors' list sizes. In my various training capacities, I have had to visit many practices and the variation was from having no waiting list right up to three weeks to have a routine appointment. This would be longer if a patient chose a particularly popular doctor in the practice, for example if there was only one lady doctor. Where there were waits, there was usually an emergency system but it was often a hassle to get through on the phone and then to persuade someone that your need was urgent.

This has been changed by a system called Advanced Access. This is a complicated replacement of the old method, unfortunately both too complicated to explain fully here and too complicated for patients to understand. In essence it means that practices are obliged to give a patient an appointment with the doctor of their choice within forty-eight hours of requesting it. To a certain extent, this works, but it is ruined by rules, the worst one being that most appointments have to be booked on the same day, making it impossible for patients or their carers to plan ahead. Many patients are very bitter about this and it is hard to say that it is an improvement.

With very few exceptions, access to GPs in most of Europe was easier than in the UK, in that appointments were always given if requested for the same day but could be booked in advance in most countries. Most of the GPs offered appointments but many did not mind if the patients walked in; indeed, in Luxembourg, where the patients have to pay to see the doctor, it is thought that offering an appointment was saving time for the patient and this convenience should and does attract a higher fee.

In Austria, patients wishing to be seen come in and pick up a ticket as at a delicatessen counter and return about two hours later to be seen. There is no appointment system in the private practice I saw in Malta and again patients walk in and pick up a number.

In countries where the pay system was mainly or totally item of service, the doctors were more consumer-orientated than here and would be more likely to see patients the same day, as the patient wanted. This was especially true of stand-alone doctors, where they were building up their practices against competition. As we have seen in Belgium, amongst other places, as patients are not registered with their doctor and can go to any doctor they choose, it is in the doctor's interest to make sure that he is freely available.

The length of the appointment was often longer than our usual ten minutes. Malta was an exception, where in the state system the routine appointment time was shorter and I was told that they can last for two to three minutes. Many of these appointments were for writing certificates or repeat prescriptions. Also in Cyprus, appointments could be as short as five minutes, depending on the case. In Slovenia, the appointment time was seven minutes. The longest, in Slovakia and Sweden, were thirty, but in most systems were twenty or fifteen.

In Sweden, however there is a waiting list for a routine appointment of three to four weeks, but they run a nurse triage system by telephone and patients will be seen the same day if necessary. These appointments are for fifteen minutes. In Finland, also, access is difficult. Getting to see a doctor in the large community health centre is like it used to be in England before Advanced Access. Patients are expected to make an appointment and it takes about two to four weeks before a patient can get to see a GP; however, there are always emergency clinics during the day and patients, if their need is urgent, can be seen on the same day. There are also triage nurses, whom patients can consult in person or by phone. The government is putting in an initiative that all urgent consultations are to be within three days. Appointment times are normally twenty minutes.

House calls are done in most countries, probably with the same variation of willingness as you would find in the UK, and like here, the rate is generallu falling. The numbers of visits that are done, and the way they are organised, vary with the doctor, the practice population as well as the country. Some doctors, as in Denmark, do as few as one visit a month. In Cyprus, they are not done at all and if the patient cannot be brought to the surgery by relatives they must go to hospital or call a private GP. In Malta, the need for house calls is reduced because doctors can send for patients in government transport.

This is a difficult area because I interviewed more than one GP in only a few countries, and although I asked them their opinion on what went on in their country as a whole, their answers must have been subjective. In most countries, either the doctor was not paid more for home visits or, if they were, the extra amount was too small to be cost effective. I found from the very beginning that I had to allow for the fact that views were often personal. For example, the doctor I interviewed in St Albans in Hertfordshire told me that he does not mind house calls, while my answer to this question would have been that I think they are a poor way of doing good medicine and should be avoided where possible.

In Austria the doctors are paid about four times the consultation rate to do a visit and their visiting rate is high by the standards of most other countries. In fact, they do about thirty in a week. In this country I saw two different GPs in different areas and I was impressed by their integrity and high ethical standards.

They both believed visiting patients at home was an important part of general practice but an outside observer cannot help wondering if the high fees have an effect on the way they see things. One of the Austrians was a single-handed country doctor and the close relationship she had with her patients may also be associated with her high visiting rate.

House calls in Finland are done only if absolutely necessary, for mainly housebound patients, and these are done by only two of seventeen doctors in the community clinic I visited. The rest of the GPs do not have to do house calls.

In France, the doctors told me the visiting rate was falling and the social security system discouraged them as they were not thought to be a good use of time. GPs who are paid partly or wholly by item of service get a higher rate for visits. In spite of this, except in Austria, these enhancements are usually too small, many told me, to be cost-effective and therefore not a good use of time. This was true even in Ireland, where the system was private and the doctors set the fees.

I have the feeling that in the Eastern European countries, which until about fifteen years ago were managed in the Soviet system, had a greater culture of visits and there has been a slow movement away from that, although in Lithuania, where visits are free of payment, it is the patients who decide if a visit is necessary and the doctor has to agree or there will be a complaint. Parents are frightened to take a sick child suffering from a mildly raised temperature out of doors. Also, having house calls saves the patient or the parent a lot of waiting around in the clinics. The GPs do about ten calls daily in winter and five in summer.

In the system in Britain, even going back fifty years, visits could in theory be only requested rather than demanded, although many doctors and all patients did not realize this. It was for the doctor, on the basis of the information given to him, to decide if a house call were necessary. In the past, many daily visits were done but the rate has been continually falling. In Latvia the patient also decides if a visit is necessary but they have to pay a small amount to see a doctor, and it is more for a visit. This may be the reason that here the GP does few, about one or two daily. However, in Estonia, where they are free, they also do about the same number.

There is a two-tier system in Slovakia which appears to be unique. The method of pay is totally by a capitation system, the sum increasing a little for patients as they get older. The doctor is allowed to charge patients for house calls if it is felt it is for social reasons and not clinically necessary. I could not find out how the distinction was made. He is also allowed to give an extra quality service, for which he charges about 150 euros a year. For this, patients have his out-of-hours number and he is willing to see them on weekends. Patients can also have visits from him, rather than the emergency service, and they can pay for this. Many patients, preferring their own doctor, accept this arrangement.

In the clinic I visited in Sweden the doctor told me it was sad but they just did not have time to do house calls. There is a central service, created for emergencies, which comes on duty at 5pm and, where possible, visits requested in the morning are left for these emergency doctors to do. By our standards, this would seem an extraordinary way to do things in that it means the visit, even when requested at a normal time will not be done by the patient's own doctor or one from the practice. Until the last couple of years, when English doctors could opt out of out-of-hours care for a small loss of income, GPs had to pay for every visit done by the out-of-hours service so this method of farming visits out would have been too expensive for GPs.

In the practice I called on in Amsterdam, the doctors did about two visits a day and, as we saw, these were done on a bicycle. The reasons for this will be obvious to anyone who has tried to drive through the centre of the city.

Telephone medicine is practiced in most places. Where there are staff acting as receptionists, calls are likely to be answered first by them and messages relayed to the doctor, who will phone back or arrange to take the call later. This is a common system and many practices use it in the UK. I regret to say that, as in this country, many doctors on the continent expect patients to phone back at a convenient time.

Other doctors do not mind being interrupted. Doctors without staff necessarily are interrupted and this depends more on the individual doctor than the system. Stand-alone doctors are more likely to be interrupted, as indeed happened several times in Belgium during our interview. In some countries, I detected a reluctance to do telephone medicine with concerns about its safety. This may be a subconscious fear developed in countries where doctors are paid for face-to-face consultations but not for those done on the phone.

In some places, such as Holland, time is set aside for patients to phone and they know when doctors are ready to receive calls. The doctors are happy to provide this facility in Holland, as it is the only country where GPs are paid to do telephone consultations and again the only place where they are paid to consult by email, although of course this position is likely to change.

Almost nowhere outside the UK were telephone consultations recorded in the notes.

When I telephoned doctors to arrange interviews, I sometimes had their mobile numbers but mostly, initially anyway, I had to phone their practice. Sometimes the doctor answered and sometimes receptionists or nurses, and we will see why when we discuss practice staff. On no occasion however did I come across an automatic switch board. These are becoming quite common here. They could be useful but in my experience, even in Barnet where I live, the way they are answered is so bad as to be embarrassing. Before you even get the list of options, you have to listen to a lecture about making sure you get your flu jab if in a designated risk group or the consequences of making but failing to keep an appointment. This is sad because British GPs are proud that they have been trained to be sensitive, yet many are not aware how it feels to have to listen to this garbage every time a patient wants a test result or a bit of advice.

Records

The use of records is different and taken much more seriously in the UK than the rest of the EU. In this country records are a very important part of medical practice, both in primary and secondary care. For this work we will study the former only.

Firstly, records allow the doctor to remember why he last saw his patient and at what stage their condition is in being solved. It is obviously important when a doctor greets his patient that he should have a reminder of why he has asked him to return and the results of any investigations in front of him. Medical records in British general practice are a complete history of all the medical events of the person's life. As someone moves away or changes doctor, his records are passed to the next practice. This has always been done by a formal arrangement, with the notes being sent to the local National Health Office which currently is the Primary Care Organization, most commonly the Primary Care Trust (PCT). These then go to the PCT of the new doctor, who sends them on to him. By this method it is possible to read about every illness noted by the GP and every letter sent by a specialist in the patient's whole life, or at least since 1948 when the National health Service (NHS) began, or sometimes even since 1911 when National Insurance began for some workers.

As will become apparent later, GPs in this country are very good at looking after chronic illnesses, such as high blood pressure and diabetes. The records on the computer are arranged so that they can be looked at in different ways. For example the doctor can look at the current notes of a patient and see how he is faring. He may have diabetes and has come to see the doctor to find out the results of his recent tests, which may result in a need to change his medication. Alternatively the doctor can use the facility that all the illnesses are arranged in lists known as 'The Disease Register'. As an example let us look at diabetes again. This illness is liable to various complications that could shorten life if neglected; these include raised blood pressure, high cholesterol and reduced kidney function. It is important therefore that these factors are measured systematically at regular intervals. It is easy for the doctor to look at his list of diabetic patients and see that most of the measurements have been done. If the success rate is not great, he can, with his team, review the practice procedures. It is important therefore that the notes are comprehensive and up to date. This system is called audit.

To enable this to happen in Britain, every medical event has to go through the NHS GP. All referrals to specialists, both NHS and private, should be done by the GP and any advice that is given or test results must be passed back to him so that the records are complete. If a heart specialist has arranged a series of follow up consultations with a patient when he measures, say, the blood pressure and cholesterol, the patient will feel no need to attend his doctor's surgery. If the results are not sent to the GP, there will be a gaping hole in the notes of this patient and he will therefore almost certainly be asked to come to the surgery to have them done, leading to a duplication of work. Mostly, these systems function well but there are some disadvantages, leading to restrictions on patients' freedoms; this is a theme that will recur in this book.

We also take accurate records seriously to protect ourselves if there is a complaint or threat of litigation. The insurance companies that protect doctors give frequent advice that it is very much easier to provide a defence if accurate and contemporary notes are available. Most doctors are aware of this and even telephone consultations are recorded.

The format could be on paper or computer. The change to electronic records, which started in the early eighties, is by now almost complete, although there are a few older doctors who still prefer paper. Letters from specialists are often scanned on to the computer so paper records are not needed at all. Arrangements are being made for the safe transmission of the letters by email. Although audit was done in the past, it has become much easier since computers were used and what used to take a whole evening's work can be done in less than five minutes.

Who owns the records? Legally of course they are the property of the PCT, but what about notionally? When I was first a medical student and I went in to the casualty department, the folders were inscribed in large letters, 'NOT TO BE HANDLED BY THE PATIENT'. By the eighties, however, we began to realize that the patient was the most important person to see the records; as he owned the illness, he should have access to what has been said about it. A law was introduced in this country that every patient has a right to demand to see his records and this must be granted unless there is a medical reason why this is harmful. In practice I have rarely found patents asking to see their records and I believe this is because we are more open with people now. I, for example, make my records on a computer and the screen is positioned in a way that the patient can read it also, although care must be taken that it is not seen by accompanying relatives and friends.

As records are such an important issue here, we must take care that making our notes on paper or computer must not intrude on the consultation. Sometimes it is possible to write them between patients but, if not, it is important not to touch the key board while the patient is speaking as this causes considerable distress. I have heard many complaints about this and have watched training videos where the computer has dominated the interview, so technique with this is very important.

Now, having described the British system and problems of record-keeping, what did I find on my travels?

As in the UK, records in Europe were advancing, frequently from being paper based to electronic, and this movement was happening at various rates, partly depending on the level of sophistication of the state systems and partly on the enthusiasm of the doctors. Extremes included Slovenia, Portugal and Cyprus where all the records are on paper and in Holland and Austria, where they seem mostly to be on computer. Both in Portugal and Cyprus computerised records are planned but development of them has not been smooth. The large health centre I visited in Lisbon had a computer in every consulting room but no software to run on them and no date for any being installed. The consulting room I saw in Nicosia, also in a large health centre, had a new computer, complete with software, installed by a Greek professor at the request of the Cypriot health authorities. Unfortunately the doctor had been given no training on how to work it so it remained unused. In many countries, where they use paper records for clinical notes, the doctors are bound by their system to use a computer connected via the internet to the authorities, to record the date and diagnosis of the consultation. This is for the purposes of pay. When I asked about confidentiality I was given different answers, in that in one country enough information had to be given that would allow the patient to be identified but in others this was not necessary.

In some places, where the records are electronic, the doctors are obliged to keep records on paper also. Slovakia is an example of this and the doctor I saw gets round this by pasting paper printouts of the consultations from the computer into the records.

There is little feeling in Europe that records should follow patients from the cradle to the grave. As we have seen, this would often not be possible because in some countries women are seen direct by primary care gynaecologists and children by primary care paediatricians. Self-referral is allowed, especially in the private sector, and the consultations are not likely to be reported to the GP. As I have shown in Finland, there are three primary care systems anyway, acting in parallel and not normally communicating with each other.

Whether or not records follow the patient is a variable feature in the EU. In some countries, this is not usual and the new doctor has to start from scratch, availing himself of the patient's history and copies of investigations that they may hold. In other countries, the records may follow the patient, either by being handed to him, or more usually the new doctor writing to the old and requesting them to be posted. I have the impression that only a proportion of doctors bother with this and it depends on goodwill. Latvia is an exception, where there is a new law by which the old doctor must send the records to the new. Although there are many different software computer systems in Belgium, by law they have to be able to talk to each other, so when a patient leaves a practice and moves elsewhere the records are sent online to the new doctor's computer. In Austria, both of the practices I visited were computerized but they had different systems which could not communicate with each other, however in this country the records are not legally required to be passed to the next doctor. Doctors in Poland are not allowed to send the records as they are required to keep them for a long period, if not indefinitely.

Patients are usually not allowed to see their records, although there are exceptions. One country, Latvia, has a law where patients can see their records but rarely use this right. In Lithuania, I am told, the patient after every consultation has to read the record and sign that it is correct.

As records seem less important in Europe they are not used so extensively as here. Although, except in Greece, most face-to-face consultations are documented, this is not common for telephone consultations. Of course, as we shall see, in those countries where the doctors have few or no staff, a telephone consultation with one patient may occur during a face-to-face consultation with another.

Target payments hardly exist in Europe, which is not surprising as there seem to be no targets. If there were, audit would be impossible because templates are rarely used, even in those rare instances where they are provided on the computer. Holland was one of the only two countries that had computers where blood pressure and similar parameters were entered into dedicated fields, making audit possible and I was told that 64 percent of GPs there use this facility. In Belgium, where computerisation varies, most doctors do use computers; the doctor I visited was able to enter all usual data in templates although audit was rarely done. In the practice I saw in Estonia, there was a comprehensive computer system with templates, but these were not used and the doctor preferred paper records anyway.

In France only some doctors have computers and there is a variety of systems. The doctor I visited does have fields for recording blood pressure and weight and these fields are used; however, there is no disease register. They cannot therefore do an audit from the computer, but audits are expected in France and are done by taking a random sample of paper records and going through those.

In fact, the only audit I came across was a diabetic audit in Holland and although general practice, as I have said, is mostly computerised, this audit is required by the health authority and is done from paper records using a random sample.

To summarise: firstly, disease registers, templates, targets and audit are not a big part of the culture of primary care in the EU outside Great Britain. Secondly, in those countries like Belgium where patients can see any GP, or those like Finland where they are likely to be seeing private GPs as well as their state ones, there is no one doctor who can be responsible to make the notes comprehensive.

Referrals

As with records, referrals seem to be taken more lightly in Europe outside the UK. We have just observed that in the UK all referrals to specialists or consultants, I use either term equally, should be done by the GP. Otherwise, unless a patient has been sent in an emergency from an Accident and Emergency department (A&E), patients will not be seen on the NHS by hospital specialists. It is considered unethical for consultants to see patients privately without referral and normally insurance companies such as BUPA and PPP have rules preventing their paying the fees if the patient was not properly referred. This rule is sometimes, however, broken because some unscrupulous consultants are willing to make a false declaration.

The advantages of such a rigid system are outlined in the description of record systems above, but the downside of loss of patients' freedom is discussed later, and the conflict produced will be considered.

Although the referral to the secondary care system in Europe is superficially similar to the UK, it is important to look at the differences. As far as I could make out, there are no objections to patients seeing private specialists privately; that is, without the state system and provided they're not expecting reimbursement. However, without the GP's letter the consultant will neither know which investigations have been done, nor the results. There is a risk therefore of their being unnecessarily repeated and they may be unpleasant, expensive or both. Similarly, he may prescribe medication which has already been tried and found to be ineffective or have unacceptable side effects.

Referral can always be made through the GP, but in many countries self-referrals are permitted even in the state systems. Again, as with private self-referral, I had the impression in these countries that there was a risk of unnecessary duplication of investigations at the state system's expense. In systems like these where, self-referral is encouraged or permitted, continuity of care must be significantly compromised. As we saw above, referral in Finland can come from any of three primary care organisations.

The view that is taken of self-referral in the state system is variable. Often there are no sanctions, although in some countries, such as Belgium, the patient gets a reduced reimbursement of the specialists' fees and in others, such as Sweden, they will have to wait longer for an appointment. At the opposite end of the spectrum, for example in Slovenia, the system is similar to ours in which GPs have a gate-keeper role and make all the referrals in the state system.

In France since 2005, with 'la réforme du médecin traitant', all patients over 16 must choose their GP, who has a new function: now he is really in charge of the patient's medical files. In the past, patients could choose freely to see whoever they wanted whenever they wanted, GPs or specialists. In this way, the GP is about to become the "gatekeeper" of medicine, as in England. Patients have a penalty in term of reimbursement if they visit a specialist without a referral from the GP they have chosen and it is the same if they decide to see a GP other than their own ('médecin traitant').

On the other end of the spectrum is Luxembourg, where patients have complete freedom and the GPs there are very proud of this. It means that, although GPs can refer patients, patients may also refer themselves to any consultant and get the same rebate. The doctors I saw did not know what proportion of patients self-refer.

No GPs I saw had secretaries to type their letters. The referrals were usually done on a prescribed form, either on paper or computer generated. The form would have fields for the patient details, problem list and medication and if on paper, these might be completed by a nurse where they exist. There was a small area on the form for the doctor to write or type what the problem was. In the UK, the majority of GPs have and use secretaries to type their referral letters and this seems to be the only country in the EU where they are usually used. Because of the general acquisition of keyboard skills in the developed world, it is likely that, as in industry, doctors here will become able to generate their own letters and rely on secretaries less.

In some countries the doctors expected and received replies and sometimes these were typed by secretaries, while in others they were typed or hand-written by the specialist. In some places these were posted and in others given to the patient. In Finland, I was told the replies came straight on-line into the patients' computerised records. In some countries, Cyprus for example, the specialists never replied to the GP's letter, and in Poland only sometimes, and GPs in these countries had to glean what information they could by seeing what investigations were done or medication prescribed.

I asked most doctors how long it would take to have a patient seen by a skin specialist and how long it would take to get a total hip replacement and, as could be imagined, the answers varied. Quite often, the waits seemed to be shorter than the in the UK, but Latvia goes to the other extreme, where a total hip operation would take 10–15 years to be completed (there must be few surviving patients who need one and are still fit for surgery). In Greece the wait is a few weeks and the idea of a waiting list for an operation of a year or two more, I am told, would cause an outcry.

Sometimes the government makes the rules but these can be bent. Finland is a typical example of this, where there is a law that a hip replacement has to be done within six months but, because there are not the resources for this, the law is used with some flexibility. Firstly, it would take a month to see the orthopaedic surgeon and then he could prevaricate by doing more investigations, such as an unnecessary MRI scan, which in itself might take months, and then eventually put the patient on the waiting list. The whole process could, in fact, take a year.

Internet Access

Broadband Internet access is provided to all GPs by the PCTs in Britain and most take advantage of it. Doctors always need information: for example, we often forget the appropriate dose of a rarely-used drug or want to make certain it is safe in pregnancy. For purposes like these we have been provided with reference books such as The British National Formulary (BNF). Now these are available on line and many of us find them much easier and faster, to look up the required information electronically. Another advantage is one can find out quickly the latest about obscure illnesses. Usually I use a medical site such as 'GP Notebook' which is a 'favourite', or sometimes I work through Google. My personal practice is to share the screen with the patient so we can study the problem together and then I can explain the relevance of what I have discovered. Many doctors work in this way.

This obviously is not available during the consultation to doctors practising in countries such as Slovenia, which still use paper records. Doctors in most countries though had computers on their desk and had internet access. There were a few exceptions, such as in Portugal, where, as stated, the computers I saw had no software and Cyprus where what I believe was the only computer in general practice had not been used. In other countries such as Germany, it is available and its use depends on the doctor. When they had it they varied as to whether they accessed information during the consultation or after but I had the feeling this was due to personal preference rather than national mores. For example both the Spanish and Italian doctors had internet on their desk and the former was happy to use it in front of patients while the latter not. Even doctors who did not have a computer on their desk could and did access the internet elsewhere, such as in an office or, as I was told by my Polish doctor, at home. As always there were idiosyncrasies and it was not always possible to know if they were personal or national. The Irish doctor told me that he and his partner do not want internet connected to their surgery computers as they fear evil people hacking into them breaching patient confidentiality.

Prescribing

There are enormous variations in the methods of prescribing, including what GPs are allowed to prescribe, how they generate their prescriptions and their methods, if any, of repeat prescribing, and the UK is no exception.

Common to nearly all the countries is the fact that patients have to contribute to the cost in some form, usually by paying a percentage of the price of the medication. If in any country the patient paid a fixed amount, this would be a maximum and if the cost of the drug were less, then that is what would be paid. In other words it seems that only in the UK, a patient being prescribed amoxicillin, a penicillin, for example, can be forced to pay a charge costing several more times the price of the medication. This is because in this country patients liable for prescription charges have to pay £6.85 for every item even though many prescriptions cost much less than that. A five day course of amoxicillin costs about £2.50. This is real 'rip-off' Britain unless, unlike me, you accept the idea that all should pay the same and the receivers of cheap medication should subsidise those who need more expensive treatment.

As well as being a rip-off, our system of prescription payments appears to have no logic to it and is roughly unchanged since it was apparently thought up by a civil servant in his bath after a heavy and liquid dinner about fifty years ago. I should point out that these charges do not apply to much of the population, including people over the age of fifty nine, children, pregnant women and various disadvantaged groups, including the chronically sick and unemployed. However, if you have one of the chronic illnesses that entitle you to be exempt from charges, then all your other conditions also become exempt. Therefore, if you have epilepsy, you do not need to pay for your asthma drugs. If your thyroid gland is under-active, you get your thyroid replacement tablets and of course medication for other illnesses. However, if your thyroid is overdoing it and you need tablets to dampen it down, that is tough, you have to pay. Probably the conditions requiring the most items of treatment are high blood pressure and asthma, but there are no exemptions there. In fact, there is no need to offer exemptions for conditions which need a larger tally of items because anyone can buy a season ticket, which is cost effective if you use more than two prescriptions a month.

In some countries there are bizarre discounts according to the illness. For example, in Poland patients pay very little towards the cost of medication for epilepsy and diabetes although there is no big discount for hypertensive medication. In Ireland, however, most patients pay the full cost of their medication as well as up to 80 euros a month for their investigations.

Prudent prescribing is encouraged in most countries in many ways. In the UK doctors are sent details of their prescribing costs and have a visit from a pharmaceutical advisor every year to discuss current prescribing issues and to suggest where GPs can choose cheaper medication without any harmful affect on treatment. In my experience, I have found these visits have been helpful and a good source of learning. For a few years they had the power to award extra payment to those doctors who met targets which they set. I did not find any system like this elsewhere.

An example of a different method of control from above is in Slovenia, where medication is free to patients but doctors prescribe from a limited list. If they go outside this list they have to justify it; if they issue drugs of limited clinical value, such as tablets to dilate peripheral arteries, they can be liable to a substantial fine. (This is about blocked arteries in the legs. It is a condition which occurs in middle age onwards and is associated with other diseases of the blood vessels including the coronary arteries. It causes intense pain in one or both calves after walking a few yards. Because the arteries are actually blocked, no drugs can dilate them, but that does not stop drug firms trying to flog them or some gullible doctors prescribing them.) In Latvia there is a list where all prescriptions carry a seventy five percent discount but the patient must pay the full cost if the doctor goes outside this list.

More common is to make the patient pay a percentage of the cost so that, as the price of a prescribed drug increases the more the patient spends, and it is hoped that there will be objections if the sum gets too high. It is not known how effective this is in limiting prescribing costs.

It is time to mention something about simvastatin here. Statins are a group of drugs which, when given continuously to patients with increased risk of having heart attacks or strokes, significantly lower these risks and are, in fact, an important medical advance. Put perhaps a little over simply they work by lowering raised cholesterol. There are many statins and although this is still controversial, there is probably little difference in the effect on the patient which one the doctor chooses. Simvastatin is the oldest and has been around so long that the patent has expired. Now any firm can make it and this has caused it to become much cheaper than any others. For this to be so, it must be prescribed generically: a problem we will come to.

The other statins, being newer, are still governed by patent and only the firms which own the patents can make them, making them much more expensive. It is therefore not a prudent use of resources to prescribe any statin other than simvastatin. Others are more potent so simvastatin will need to be given in a higher dose, but still the price advantage remains. I found it interesting to see the variation between countries when dealing with this issue.

It is a common phenomenon that when statins are used GPs are confined to Simvastatin; in Slovakia, the dose prescribed by GPs is limited to 20mg daily and if a higher amount or a different preparation is indicated the patient must be referred to a consultant clinic. In Germany, the limited list again includes only simvastatin and if either doctor or patient prefers a different one either can choose to pay the extra cost; I was not surprised to be told it is unlikely that doctors would agree to this, although the patient might. Cyprus is another country where the only statin GPs can use is simvastatin and here the antibiotics they can choose also come from a limited choice. I shall have more to say on antibiotic prescribing later. Also, the only modern antidepressant they are allowed to use themselves is Seroxat. Holland limits its prescribing bill to a certain extent by expecting patients to buy over the counter 'bathroom cabinet' drugs such as laxatives, antacids, antihistamines and painkillers.

As with simvastatin, the patent on other drugs runs out in time, making them cheaper as other firms produce them. A common dodge is for their original manufacturer to bring out a replica with a similar name and a slightly altered molecule but no discernible clinical difference. They then tell foolish doctors that this is even better than there were making before and of course they have a fresh patent on the new one. This problem is often ignored but in England the pharmaceutical advisor will explain the pointlessness of prescribing these new ones and in Slovakia these medications, described as of limited clinical value, are not allowed.

Generic prescribing is a hot issue, raising strong feelings. A generic prescription is where the name of the drug is the one given rather than that chosen by the manufacturer. Analogies would be saying vacuum cleaner rather than Hoover or ball point pen rather than Biro. As I hope is becoming clear, the cost is the same for those medications if the patent has not run out, but for the rest the difference is important. I have a copy of the British National Formulary (BNF) in front of me. I find that a packet of thirty Prozac capsules, each of twenty milligrams, is priced at £14.21. However if Fluoxetine, which is what Prozac is, is prescribed, the price is £1.56. It is clear therefore that doctors have the power to cause a ridiculous waste of national health money in many countries.

Although generic prescribing is usually encouraged, or even demanded by the state authorities, doctors in some countries hate

157

it, while others approve. Although encouraged, so far it has reached only a ten percent level in Portugal and thirty percent in Belgium, for example. In the UK it is eighty three percent. Many doctors do not trust the quality of the preparations and feel they are giving their patient inferior treatment. The doctor I saw in Italy thought that generic preparations could be fake and therefore tended to avoid them, and although I was not sure if her views were general, I had the impression that what most doctors told me about generic prescribing was common for their country. Many patients, even those who are paying, insist on branded drugs, which cost them more. I was told that consultants in some countries try and insist on the use of branded drugs, possibly, as one cynic told me, because they are hosted with all expenses paid at international conferences. There is no choice, however, in Holland where the GPs have to prescribe generically; if they don't, the pharmacist is obliged to substitute the prescription for a generic one.

In the UK when a doctor issues a generic prescription, he has no power to choose which company will make it. However in some countries, including Belgium, when a doctor prescribes generically, he can also name the manufacturer, for example *Amoxicillin-Sandoz*.

There is another, rather semantic, confusion in comparing the rates of generic prescribing by country, and this is how to classify a drug that is still on patent. Here, if we use the generic name, it is counted as generic prescribing. However, it was pointed out to me in Spain that, regardless of what is written, if the drug is in patent, the patient can get only the branded drug; so generic prescribing in this circumstance is meaningless.

Author's digression on generic prescribing.

From my travels I have learnt that the UK is one of the countries most keen on generic prescribing, giving doctors a lot of pressure but also some rewards. I have always thought this was the right thing to do as it saves a lot of money and there is no evidence that there is any clinical difference. Because of this I have always been proud of my own practice which has continually had the highest level of generic prescribing in Barnet and was known as a Beacon Practice.

However, apart from pecuniary considerations, it comes at a severe cost. It seems that the companies that make the tablets can call them what they like, put them in different packaging, with different names and give the tablets any old appearance. For example, two common treatments for high blood pressure are atenolol and amlodipine. Atenolol, as well as coming in various boxes, is usually round, but can come in cream or bright orange colours, among others. Amlodipine comes in all sorts of containers and the tablets vary from small round disks to small white lozenge shaped objects. It does not take a lot of thought to realize the concern this causes, especially for patients with high blood pressure, diabetes and angina who may be taking, quite reasonably, over ten different daily preparations. These are sometimes laid out into special containers with a month's supply where each day's dose is counted out. Sometimes circumstances change when a medication or dose needs to be changed during the month and imagine the distress of the patient or their carer when this happens.

If, as we should, we are going to help the economy by using generic prescribing, where possible our patients and we have the right to expect that the government does what it can to remove any difficulties. This should be done by their insisting on uniform presentation of tablets, including their names and packaging, before licensing firms make these drugs at the National Health's expense. We now even have this sort of abuse with proprietary prescribing. As has been emphasized one of the most contentious issues is whether any statin other than Simvastatin should normally be used. In March 2005, for example, twenty-eight tablets of twenty milligrams cost £7.80, while twenty-eight tablets of ten milligrams of Atorvastatin, which is an equivalent dose, was £18.03. It is very doubtful, although controversial, that there is any clinical benefit of one over the other. In the UK the makers call it 'Lipitor' and this name seems to be used in much of Europe. However, for the same price, chemists are dispensing an Atorvastatin (By the same makers) called 'Tahore' so even at this exorbitant cost patients are not being given the security of a familiar name. It seems that in this respect our NHS controllers have lost all control over what is going on.

While on the subject of prescribing anomalies, there is another nonsense I must mention. To save wasting money we are exhorted to limit our prescribed quantities to a month at a time. However, the governenment, who pays for most of this medication, has not defined what a month is, and some *tablets are made in boxes of twenty eight and others in thirty, causing confusion for doctors and patients and annoyance for pharmacists.*

In most countries GPs, are allowed to prescribe a full range of drugs with few exceptions, such as specialist cancer drugs. Unless you believe that GPs should not have the same power to choose as hospital doctors, there are worrying exceptions to this. In the state system in Malta, for example, GPs are obliged to continue what the consultant has started, even if they do not agree with it. They are limited as to which statins they are allowed to choose and are not allowed to prescribe them at all unless the bad cholesterol is above a certain level. GPs are also degraded in Lithuania where, when a GP diagnoses a disease like diabetes, he is bound to refer the patient to a specialist to confirm the diagnosis. The specialist will start or suggest a treatment which the GP must prescribe. The patient must be seen at regular intervals, depending on the case, for the GP to be allowed to continue to prescribe. Other illnesses in this category include chronic heart disease and treatment for an enlarged prostate gland. If a patient with high blood pressure had a heart attack and had not been seen by a specialist for some years, the GP would be in some sort of trouble.

In Greece, prescribing medication for psychological illness is made difficult, apart from fluoxetine which is of course Prozac. For everything else, such as Valium or a sleeping tablet, the prescription has to start with a special note from the internist. The patient has to take that to the municipal authorities and a doctor there will read what the internist has written and write the prescription on a special form with a red line down the front. Only then can a pharmacist dispense it.

There are strict rules for treating depression by GPs in Slovenia, which are taken seriously because it is thought that it is the country with the third highest suicide rate in the world, Hungary being the first. The rules are that if the patient has any question of psychotic illness, they fail to respond to three different antidepressants, or if they appear to be suicidal, they have to be referred to a psychiatrist. As well as using antidepressants, GPs, if trained, will try and give the patient counselling and there are counsellors and cognitive behaviour therapists to whom they can refer their patients.

160

Repeat prescribing systems vary. Some countries can give a repeating prescription, for example, as in France and Latvia, one that will enable the pharmacist to dispense one month and then repeat this for up to six months; while in Sweden, a prescription can authorize the pharmacist to dispense three months' supply at a time, up to one year. In other countries, repeat prescriptions are not allowed and in those where the maximum amount is limited to one to three months, the patient must return to the surgery. In some systems, they are forced to have a face-to face consultation with the doctor, generating more income for some, such as in Austria, but not of course in countries where doctors are salaried.

I have written above that in Germany there is a peculiar capitation pay system where a patient must be seen at least once every three months to stay on the list and therefore for the doctor to be paid. This means that a prescription will never be for a supply that lasts longer than three months, as the doctor needs the patient to return in this period for another consultation.

In other countries, GPs, instead of using a repeat prescribing system, where there are no limits to what they can give, will issue a prescription for six months supply at a time, and the patient will buy what they need in installments.

I usually asked if it was necessary for consultations to end in a prescription. I was not surprised to discover that there was a wide range of answers. The Spanish GP was an experienced trainer and gave the same answer as I would have done, in that he usually felt it always necessary to prescribe in his youth but with increasing experience he has, when medication is not likely to be helpful, been able to convince the patient of this, whilst allowing him to feel his illness is not being neglected. However, where the practices are mostly independent, doctors told me that, although they should not usually finish with prescriptions, they tend to lose patients if they do not issue some medication, and as shown below this has an effect on antibiotic prescribing rates.

I asked about antibiotic prescribing. The problems here can be simply put. Antibiotics are effective in bacterial disease but not in viral. Pneumonia, an infection of the lungs, is usually bacterial and it responds well to antibiotics. It causes a cough and fever and these tend to get better quickly. Unfortunately most coughs and fevers come from colds or flu, which are viral infections and cannot possibly respond to antibiotics. In fact, there is probably no medicine which has any beneficial effect on these conditions and, what makes it worse, the coughs can go on unabated for weeks or months causing considerable distress but no risk to the sufferers and, if children, their parents. Doctors, being kind people and also hating to have nothing useful to offer, have not always understood this and prescribed antibiotics for coughs and colds. Even when the lungs sound fine up the stethoscope they kid themselves because the phlegm is green that there is a 'chest infection', truly a non-existent condition. If the illness gets better coincidentally at the same time, it is natural that the patient will see it as cause and effect and expect the same treatment for every recurrence. There are many examples of when antibiotics may or may not be needed but what are called Upper Respiratory Tract Infections (URTIs), in other words, coughs and colds, cause the greatest amount of useless antibiotic prescribing.

Almost every doctor I spoke to was aware that there was a history of over-use of these preparations and efforts were or should be being made to do something about it. As expected, there was a varying degree of success. Every doctor and many patients know that if antibiotics are widely used, the bacteria in the community will become resistant to them. As it happens, outside hospitals in the UK, most bacteria are still sensitive to the antibiotics invented a long time ago, which are now of course cheap. These are known as 'first line'. These are usually penicillins, the most popular ones being known as Penicillin V and Amoxicillin. There are new and expensive antibiotics, called reasonably "second line", which, when used to treat bacterial infection which has become resistant to an old preparation, can be effective and even life saving. They are rarely needed and, to preserve their effectiveness and also to avoid wasting money, they should be used with care. Over-use of these in England, when it occurs, is regularly discussed in the annual visit by the prescribing advisor.

Although in many places the use of antibiotics had fallen, some doctors, such as those in Portugal, told me that the rates of prescribing in their country were far too high and would take a long time to get better. In Greece, the rate of use, although very high, is falling partly because demand will not necessarily generate a prescription for antibiotics, particularly in the health centres, where the doctors have nothing to lose if a patient is not happy. In Austria, in the country, where there were a lot of foreign workers, I was told it was more difficult to explain to them why antibiotics were unnecessary.

I learnt that in Luxembourg and France antibiotics were over-used but efforts to educate doctors and patients were showing positive results.

In Finland, the position is improving and they believed that they would find themselves in the middle of a European league table for antibiotic prescribing, although the first choice in the health centre which I visited was Azithromycin. This is one of a group known as macrolides and, except when patients are allergic to penicillin, is considered as second line. They tend to be expensive in the UK.

There are problems in Eastern European countries where many GPs, as we have seen, have recently taken over their practices as a business from state control and are trying to build them up. In these circumstances it is thought that refusing antibiotics will cause the patient to change doctors. However I was told in Latvia that they are used responsibly.

In Lithuania and Estonia they use the 'delayed' system, which is becoming popular over here. If a patient has what appears to be a viral infection, such as a cough, they will be given a prescription for antibiotics and advised to wait two or three days to see if they need it. Writing for myself, I have never seen the advantage of this method of prescribing. If, clinically, a cough is thought to be caused by a virus the diagnosis will not change in three days. It is obvious, I hope, from what I said above that the problem is a psycho-social one. It is very hard for doctors to refuse to prescribe antibiotics when a patient is racked by a persistent cough and has expectations that he will be prescribed them. It is difficult for the doctor to withhold them under these circumstances, especially as there is no other useful treatment. GPs have to learn consultation skills so that they can make it clear that they understand their patient's suffering and share the distress that nothing can be done, and yet have the consultation ending with the patient understanding, and being satisfied with, the doctor's care.

In Italy, I learnt that antibiotics are used a lot. Patients have a high expectation of being given antibiotics and there is a feeling that first line ones are not effective and second line ones are often used, although the GP I saw is concerned this may be dangerous. This was quite a common response to my questions about antibiotics. In some countries it appears that Penicillin V and Amoxicillin are hardly used any longer. Also, in Portugal there is concern that second line antibiotics are inappropriately used. However, as we have seen in Cyprus, only specialists are allowed to prescribe second line ones. Where antibiotics are over-prescribed or where the initial choices are second line ones, the doctors are aware of the issues and put it down to patient demand. This use of second line preparations has led in Spain to a feeling by doctors that Amoxicillin is not effective and therefore can be used as a placebo in patients who inappropriately demand antibiotics.

Sweden, Holland and Belgium are proud of their record of being low on the table of use of antibiotics and GPs use them responsibly. The doctors do not prescribe antibiotics for viral infections and when antibiotics are used, they use first line ones, mostly Penicillin V.

Mostly, however, there were improvements and these had usually occurred through improving doctor and patient education, as in the UK. However, in one country, I was told that a reason for improvement in the quantity of antibiotics issued was due to the fact that they used to be available over the counter. This has now stopped, leading to a change of culture.

Investigations

For a doctor to make a diagnosis, as well as taking a history and making a relevant examination, it is often necessary to do some investigations. Even when looking after well people in the performance of health promotion some tests, such as cholesterol, are necessary. Most tests fall into one of two categories: those measuring things in blood and urine, and those involving imaging, which means x-rays and scans. Mostly in the UK GPs have the same rights to arrange tests as consultants, although there are exceptions with expensive types of scans such as Magnetic Resonance Imaging (MRI) scans.

In the past, in the UK, phlebotomy, the process of taking blood from the patient, could have been done at the hospital where the laboratory is, although many doctors took the blood themselves. Later, when practice nurses were employed, this was one of their assigned roles. Eventually the nurses came under too much pressure as they took on other more sophisticated tasks and this service was no longer offered routinely. Some PCTs arrange for hospital phlebotomists (technicians who are trained to take blood but nothing else clinical) to attend surgeries once a week and the rest of the time the patient will have to go to the hospital to get the test done. If, of course, they drive to the hospital, they will have to pay for parking, sometimes up to four pounds, which means the NHS is no longer free at the point of delivery. I did not come across this problem anywhere else, in that if there were nurses in a practice who

165

could take blood, they would do it regardless of their other duties. It varied as to whether patients had their phlebotomy done in the practice or in a laboratory.

Mostly throughout Europe doctors have a similar range of investigations to those in the United Kingdom. There is variation, however, on whether the patients pay, with or without a rebate, or if it is totally free. In Poland, however, the GP pays for the investigations out of his capitation fee, which allows for this. Therefore, if he needs to refer a patient to a specialist he is expected to do the preliminary investigations. He would expect the consultants, while the patient is under their care, to do further investigations, thus avoiding the GP the expense. These would include MRI scans and other advanced imaging tests which are usually ordered by specialists, and GPs cannot arrange these there. Ultra-sound of the abdomen is provided by GPs. Specialists and GPs have their own list of tests which each are supposed to run in their office. There does not seem to be any holding back on investigations by GPs to save themselves money.

In some countries, the GPs actually do some of their own investigations and own auto-analysers which, as the name implies, automatically do the required tests. They are expensive and cannot do all necessary investigations, but do a useful amount. They are paid an item of service for each test. Austria is an example of this. The doctor I met there owns an auto-analyser and is paid by the state for all investigations he does in his practice with it. For the more sophisticated tests, he has to send the blood to a laboratory which, of course, is paid for those.

There is variation in how the results come to the GP. As expected, where doctors have computers the results may go into them direct. In many practices in the UK now, the results come via an email line direct from the laboratory to the patients' computerised records, although the GP would study these daily before they are electronically filed. If the practice is not fully computerised, or the laboratory is still developing, the results come on paper. In the practices I saw in Madrid and Rome, the results come in on paper and are entered into the computer. One doctor told me that he uses two laboratories, one of which posts the results on paper, while the other sends them electronically, and he prefers the former.

In some places the patients are given a choice of where they have their blood tests. In Luxembourg, the GP told me that he uses a whole series of laboratories, depending entirely on patients' choice. Some patients prefer to have their investigations near work, others near their home. Some go to hospitals and some go to private clinics, but none have to pay. He does not mind the fact that the results come back on various different pieces of paper and faxes. This is one of many examples where Luxembourg seems to me to be more consumer-orientated than elsewhere. A few other countries had a similar range of laboratories.

In Belgium, where as we shall see later, they work without staff, the doctor I met can provide a complete range of investigations and for some patients he takes the bloods himself, whilst the laboratory does it for the rest. For the ones that he takes, the laboratory sends a car to pick up the specimens. The results come down on to his computer at 6pm. He is required to keep paper records of the investigations.

There are curious exceptions and limitations to the range of investigations available. In Malta, the doctors cannot arrange thyroid function tests, so thyroid illness is investigated and managed entirely in secondary care. In Britain, as in most other countries, thyroid disease is normally investigated and treated by GPs, and only complicated cases need to be referred. Elsewhere, because testing for glycosolated haemoglobin (HBA1C) is expensive and thought to be unnecessary, it is not available to GPs, and diabetes has to be managed only by reference to blood glucose. The HBA1C is usually thought to be a most important test in the management of diabetes, to the extent that it would be difficult to know how a patient is doing without it. In practice, if this test is not available to GPs, the patient would have to be managed at hospital, which is a pity as GPs should be trained to look after this disease to a high standard. I should qualify this statement by pointing out that there are two types of diabetes known as Type l and Type ll. Roughly speaking, the former need insulin while the latter do not. Insulin-dependent diabetics form a small proportion of the whole and these usually need the care of specialists but the Type ll cases can and should be managed in primary care.

General practitioners in Lithuania are expected to own equipment and do their own investigations, including full blood count, creatinine (which is a measure of kidney function, liable to be affected in chronic illnesses such as high blood pressure and diabetes), cholesterol, blood sugar and urine analysis. They are not paid extra for this; it is just part of the work they are supposed to do, and, as in Poland, the cost is included in their capitation fee. For any further investigations, including HBA1C, they would be expected to refer patients to the hospital, where the specialist would arrange it. If a GP wishes to do further investigations himself, he can do so, but then the patient must pay. This seems to act as a big deterrent to GPs to investigate their patients fully and seems rather degrading for them compared with consultants.

European GPs normally have no difficulties arranging imaging. They can refer patients for a full range of x-rays, except in Malta where in the state sector they can arrange chest x-rays, but not abdominal x-rays; they cannot arrange any x-rays to see if there has been a fracture but must refer to trauma specialists. They can order all tests in a private laboratory or radiology clinic and private doctors have an ultrasound unit in their practice, but then the patient has to pay. Usually, there was no delay in fixing ultrasound scans, although Cyprus was an exception and I was told that, there it can take up to three months. There was more variation in getting computerised tomography (CT) scans and MRI scans. CT scans are cheaper than MRI scans but in many conditions do not show as much useful information. Mostly, the patient had to be referred to a specialist but sometimes, as in Slovakia, a word on the phone would be enough. In Germany the GP can arrange CT and MRI scans himself but the insurance company would expect him to justify the expense with compelling clinical reasons. In Finland, although patients must be referred for CT and MRI scans, the waiting lists for these are about a week and not as expensive as in other countries because there is a list of providers who compete with each other. In the UK the position regarding MRI scans varies; until recently in the Barnet PCT, where I work, GPs had to refer the requests to specialists and there were long waits. Recently, as in Finland, our PCT has contracted this service to a private organization and the GPs can refer direct with a shorter wait. Not only are the MRI scans cheaper for the PCT but also they do not have to pay for expensive consultant appointments.

In summary, in most but not all countries, general practitioners can organize the same blood tests that we can. However, for the patient they are more likely to have their phlebotomy done on site. Where practices employ nurses or a form of health care assistant who can take blood, they would do so and see it as part of their duties. In these practices, patients would not have to wait for a few days or weeks or be referred to the laboratory for phlebotomy. Where GPs work in clinics with primary care gynaecologists, there is likely to be ultrasound equipment on site. This is because gynaecologists also act as obstetricians (doctors who are in charge of pregnancy and delivering babies), and have more need of ultrasound than most. Equipment on site is more likely to be cost-effective for them.

Health Promotion

Health promotion is the other half of medicine. Traditionally doctors have been there for people who feel ill and they want someone trained to find out what is wrong and if possible to make them better. Health promotion is a concept which allows people who feel well to discover if things are about to go wrong and take action to put them right. Some of health promotion is to detect cancer before there are any symptoms, so it can be dealt with at an early stage when treatment is more likely to be effective.

Probably the largest part of health promotion at present is detecting the risk factors for cardio-vascular disease (CVD). This group of illnesses, which includes heart attacks, strokes and poor blood supply in the legs, leading to pain on walking, and (rarely) gangrene, leads to more premature deaths and illness even than cancer. The risk factors for CVD are many and mostly do not have symptoms. These include high blood pressure and Type ll Diabetes, which usually has no symptoms in the early stages and yet poses a serious risk of CVD and raised cholesterol. The object of health promotion is to discover these factors and do something about them.

Another task of health promotion is to encourage a healthy life style. There is conclusive evidence that lack of exercise and obesity contribute to the prevalence of CVD and smoking is one of the most serious risk factors, not only for CVD but also for cancer of the lungs and, one of the worst of all, what used to be called chronic bronchitis and emphysema, but has been renamed Chronic Obstructive Respiratory Disease (COPD).

Health promotion is something which can be done only systematically and we have been good at this in the UK for some years. Many practices realized the importance of this and set targets in which they would get the blood pressure of all their adult patients measured at regular intervals. If it was raised they, would not only treat it to a given level but search for the other risk factors as well when indicated. They kept disease registers of all serious conditions like diabetes and raised blood pressure and studied them at regular intervals to make sure they were reaching their target of a high percentage of patients having their risk factors under control. Until 2004, there was no extra payment for this and only some doctors were doing it comprehensively. Because of this, a new contract was introduced by which doctors were paid if they reached targets set by the government who, through the PCTs, send in inspectors to do the audits.

Because of all this, there should be a significant fall in the rates of premature death from CVD in Britain and, indeed, this is happening. There are three disadvantages. Firstly, it turns healthy citizens into patients, who often have to be persuaded to take several tablets, even though they feel well. Secondly, it can interfere with a consultation. For example, a patient can come to see his GP with pain in a knee and may hope to mention, if the doctor appeared in a friendly mood that he was depressed. He now has to fit all this in with the doctor's agenda which could mean that he needs to check the blood pressure if it has not been done for more than three years and have a discussion about his smoking. Lastly, the system can work well only if the GP has all the records, so the patient is tied to the practice. We will come to this when looking at the conclusions at the end.

Health promotion is usually done opportunistically. This means that when the patient attends the surgery with his own agenda, the doctor or the nurse will use the opportunity to check their blood pressure. Nearly all people see their doctor at least once every three years, so these opportunities are important. Once a condition is diagnosed and treated, the patient will need to return regularly for his medication.

Now let us look at what I found on the continent. This subject, if tackled at all is approached in a variety of ways, with a range of formality. In Slovenia, for example there are quite stringent arrangements for health promotion. The doctors are required to make sure that every patient has a blood pressure check every year, no matter what the age is and because these blood pressure recordings are not on computer, they have to check the records every time. It is quite permissible, however, for the blood pressure to be checked by the nurse. On top of this, men over the age of 35 and women over the age of 40, assuming they have normal blood pressure, have to have a three-year cardio-vascular check, which includes measuring the blood glucose and cholesterol.

Many doctors told me they do health promotion opportunistically, such as taking the BP at each attendance and some had nurses to do it for them each time (see under *Staff Including Nurses* below). No one was able to audit this, so their success rate was unknown. A doctor I interviewed in Austria told me he will record blood pressure opportunistically and so he, believes, do pharmacists. I did not find out if pharmacists were ever used systematically for this purpose in Austria or elsewhere.

The Belgian doctor I met takes blood pressure opportunistically and in almost every consultation. This is partly due to the fact that his consultations, even follow-ups, last for twenty-five minutes. He is not sure whether this is done in other parts of Belgium. There are no other forms of regular health promotion.

There are various plans for health promotion in Holland, where many doctors try to take blood pressure opportunistically. However, as there is no template for this they have to look through the records to see when it was last done. There is also a 'stop smoking' programme to be used whenever a doctor sees a patient who admits smoking. In addition, against influenza, every person at risk is vaccinated. A cervical screening programme is also done by GPs in co-operation with public health care organizations. Finally, there is a protocol for the identification and treatment of patients with a higher than normal risk for cardiovascular diseases.

In the Czech Republic, adults are invited for a check-up to be done by the doctor every two years. As well as blood pressure measurement and weight, a physical examination is done including chest and abdomen. I was rather surprised at this because routine examinations of the chest and abdomen are not likely to lead to the discovery of many previously undiagnosed and treatable conditions. Although the pick-up rate is minimal, there are no complaints by the doctors as they are well paid for this. Also cholesterol and Prostate Specific Antigen (PSA) are measured at prescribed times. The PSA is a marker for the presence of cancer of the prostate.

Curiously, in Poland, not every doctor offers health promotion and any GP can do it on any patient, not necessarily his own. Doctors are paid separately for this. The results are given in writing to the patient and, if abnormal, he is encouraged to take these to his regular GP. There is no procedure in place to see that this is done. If urgent action is required, such as referral to secondary care, the doctor doing the health promotion will do that. However, the Polish system is quite comprehensive. Over the age of twenty-five, patients are encouraged to make regular health promotion visits and these consist of a blood pressure check, a lipid (this is mainly cholesterol) measurement and a fasting blood glucose. This is done every three years. Additionally there is a programme to prevent cancer of the colon. The idea is that people who are going to get this cancer have risk factors that could lead to their developing this condition one day and an examination of the bowel (colonoscopy) will discover it while it is still in a curable stage. Therefore, between the ages of forty and sixty-five, during the health promotion interview, the patient is asked about abdominal pain, bowel habit, loss of weight, blood in the stools and family history of cancer. Every bit of this risk stratification has points and if a certain number of points are reached, the patient is referred for a routine colonoscopy. There are other ways for screening for this cancer including testing the stool for traces of blood. The whole subject is still being debated.

In Lithuania and Latvia, certain employees have to have a health check at regular intervals. This would include, for example, teachers and people working at computers who would need an eye check, tree surgeons who would need to be checked for psychological fitness so they will not throw themselves off; and other occupations also give rise to appropriate examinations.

There is no specific health promotion system in Cyprus or Estonia, but many patients, especially women in the latter, continually ask for their blood pressure and cholesterol to be measured. In Sweden and Denmark, if this is done at all, it is on an opportunistic basis as there are no routine plans for regular blood pressure checking or blood tests. I mentioned the Finnish system earlier, where, it will be remembered, there is a comprehensive occupational health scheme in which sometimes the occupational health physicians give primary care. People would have to be employed to obtain these health promotion services. The system seems to mean that the employed staff in the community health centre has systematic health promotion but not necessarily their patients unless they are working.

These notes mention only a few countries as it was quite common for me to be told that the country that I was in had no arrangements for health promotion at all, although some had something pending. These remarks do not include cervical cytology, as outside the UK this is not usually seen to be the responsibility of the GP.

Enthusiasm for smoking cessation seems to depend on a combination of the arrangements of a country and the feelings of particular doctors. Only rarely are there smoking cessation clinics, Cyprus being an exception, although the doctor I saw in Estonia had been on a smoking cessation course. It is not usual in Europe for free patches and other anti-smoking medication to be provided.

The problems of smoking are compounded where many doctors smoke and I was told that in Greece the smoking rate for doctors is thirty-eight percent, while in Hungary about eighty percent smoked. It is also high in some other countries. In Slovenia the problem is that, although few doctors smoke, this is not true of nurses.

Doctors in Denmark have a general feeling that they should discourage patients from smoking, but it does not seem to be as big an issue as it is in the UK. Few doctors smoke there.

Dutch general practice has a very strong smoking cessation policy. The doctors have had a considerable amount of training in smoking cessation and they have a programme to counsel patients and advise them how to obtain patches or tablets. It will be remembered that GPs in Holland are paid for each consultation as well as capitation fees and are allowed to charge the equivalent of three consultations together for a smoking cessation session. There is also a strong smoking cessation policy in Belgium. It is not necessarily or even usually run by GPs, but any suitable citizen who has had a year's training can become a Master of Tabak and patients are referred by GPs to these masters for treatment.

Smoking cessation does not appear to be related to policy about smoking in public places. For example, Italy was one of the first countries to ban smoking in restaurants, yet there appears to be no smoking cessation policy, no prescription of patches or other drugs and no smoking cessation clinics. Many Italian doctors smoke. Conversely, in the UK there was a comprehensive smoking cessation policy in place, with incentives for the doctors, free prescriptions and clinics, long before the problems of smoking in public places was tackled. Poland is similar to the UK in this respect, in that GPs are encouraged to persuade patients to give up smoking and they can refer patients to a smoking cessation clinic, although they do not prescribe patches. I was told that only a few GPs smoke in Poland and as far as I know there are no laws planned to stop smoking in restaurants.

The doctor I saw in Malta told me that although he appreciates smoking is not good for health, he thinks that smoking cessation clinics are effective only if patients want to stop, and he does not badger patients to stop smoking at every visit, although he does prescribe patches and tablets (Zyban) to motivated patients.

Guidelines

Many years ago doctors treated illness in the way they thought best. The trouble was that many thought differently from each other and, therefore, the treatment that the patient was given depended more on the doctor than the illness. Over the last forty years groups of doctors have used scientific methods to examine which treatment gives the best result and published their findings. The results are known as guidelines and an increasing number of doctors are happy to work from these, as they are likely to give the best care that is known.

In the UK, many illnesses or organs such as the heart have their own groups studying treatment. There is the British Hypertension Society for high blood pressure and the British Cardiac Society for heart disease. These are just two examples but there are many others. Much research is studied by the specialists before they produce their guidelines, and these are published in peer reviewed journals. Also guidelines are produced by NICE and some are used in the QOF requirements. Fortunately, the varying sources of guidelines do show a large measure of consistency.

Before looking at how they are used in the rest of Europe I would like to give an example of a topical set of guidelines when treating raised cholesterol. It is generally accepted that high cholesterol is bad, in that it is an important risk factor for CVD. As it would be too expensive for everyone to take statins and, anyway, there could be side effects, it seems sensible to work out who are the people who are most likely to benefit from them. It has been generally agreed to divide the issue into secondary prevention and primary prevention of CVD. The former is easy. Patients who has have any CVD illness in the past, including heart attacks, angina and strokes, together with all diabetics, are considered at increased risk and should have a statin. The latter is more complicated. The art of primary prevention is to determine which apparently healthy patients have enough risk factors to have something to gain from it. The system used is risk stratification, and this weighs several factors including gender, age, whether a current smoker, the level of the blood pressure before treatment and how much of the total cholesterol is good cholesterol, known as High Density Lipoprotein (HDL). It is not necessary to discuss HDL any further here, except to say that the higher the level of it the better, and there is often a lot of it in women, making it unnecessary to treat their cholesterol in primary prevention. Use of risk stratification is part of our guidelines. The risk stratification is usually done either on a special computer program or user friendly charts. In many practices, including my own, there are large laminated charts on each doctor's desk.

Guidelines in other European countries are used in many different ways, but not usually as formally as in the UK. Some countries, including Germany, Hungary and Austria, have their own, although there seems to be no pressure to use them; some countries use the guidelines prepared by other countries. For example, the Irish doctor I met uses UK and Scottish ones while in Slovenia they use Finnish ones, which are currently being translated into Slovene. Others rely on international guidelines. As in many countries where doctors work on their own, they tell me they use guidelines but have no means of knowing whether their colleagues do.

As we have seen, when looking at health promotion, because of the almost universal lack of targets, templates and audits, it is very difficult to know what is done in the way of keeping to guidelines, although most doctors claim to be using something. It is usually impossible, without audits, to discover how many patients with risk factors or chronic disease have their blood pressure or cholesterol controlled or are taking aspirin. The doctor in Spain who worked in a group practice of fourteen doctors is very experienced and he told me sadly that for three years he did monthly audits for his whole practice but was disappointed to find no improvements and was persuaded by his colleagues to desist.

In Denmark I was told that there are local and international guidelines. It is not clear how much these are used, for example; statins are prescribed for secondary prevention, but there seems to be little use of statins in primary prevention and no risk stratification.

However, in Belgium there are national guidelines and these and international guidelines are quite clearly used. There is differentiation between primary and secondary prevention of raised cholesterol and in primary prevention they use the similar risk stratification to that which we do in the UK, the difference being that they have to justify to the health authority that they have done this before being allowed to prescribe statins.

France is also taking guidelines seriously. The doctor I met was working part-time for the Change to Haute Autorité de Santé (HAS) organisation which is producing national guidelines for France, similar to the NICE guidelines in the UK; however, there are some difficulties in implementing these guidelines. Since July 1st 2005, all doctors (GPs and specialists) have been obliged to make an assessment of their professional activity, called 'Évaluation des pratiques professionnelles' (EPP). This assessment has to be done on the basis of guidelines. At the present time, HAS is making a great effort to incite doctors to use guidelines in order to improve their practice.

Some countries, such as Malta, do not allow the GPs to have guidelines, as all management is laid down by specialists with the GPs blindly following.

The doctor in Estonia told me that in her country, doctors work from usual international guidelines, and the treatment for hypertension seems to be conventional. It is not quite clear to me under what circumstances statins are used. There does not seem to be a rigid separation of primary and secondary prevention, nor a fixed system of risk stratification. Patients are more likely to have statins if their blood pressure is raised, but not if they smoke. This was the response I had in several countries.

In other places, such as Cyprus, I was told that there are no practice guidelines. All doctors are free to work exactly as they like. However, discussions with the GP about chronic disease management, including risk factors for CVD, show that their work is quite conventional by our standards.

As we saw under *Money Matters* above, doctors in Holland are paid to run a diabetic programme.

As noted in *Prescribing* above, there are strict guidelines for treating depression in Slovenia.

As with health promotion, I came away with the impression that our systematic and audited use of guidelines makes us the most advanced country in Europe in the detection and treatment of chronic disease. However well doctors in other countries do, because of the rare use of templates and therefore the lack of audits, they are not able to tell how they are doing and make the necessary changes. The countries who come nearest are Holland and Belgium, who at least have the facilities for audit on their computers, even if at present they are not used.

Alternative Medicine

Mostly I found in Europe the view of GPs varied but there was a similar range to the UK. That is, most doctors prefer to have little to do with it, with a few getting angry at its being used, especially by qualified doctors, and a few at the other end of the scale supporting it and even doing it themselves. In fact, the doctor I visited for this project in England, working in a group practice, is a strong supporter of acupuncture, which he practises free on his practice NHS patients, and also earns money by doing this for private patients. On balance, it seemed that throughout the continent the doctors were less than enthusiastic and not at all interested in the subject, but there were extremes. The usual response was that, although not encouraged, it is allowed, but the health service will not pay for it (except, where applicable, a usual consultation fee) and, with exceptions, the doctors cannot charge patients for it, except in countries like the UK and Denmark, where they can charge other doctors' patients for it.

When doctors qualify in Slovenia they have to sign an undertaking that they are not going to do alternative or complementary medicine, otherwise they cannot obtain a licence to practise conventional medicine. This, however, was an exception.

I was told in Sweden that there doctors prefer evidence-based medicine and are required by law to practise according to "science and acknowledged experience".

Germany is different in that some doctors practise homeopathy and complementary medicine, although if they do this it is normal for them to have some qualification in this field. The health insurance agency does not pay them for alternative medicine, but the doctor is allowed to charge the patient direct.

In Holland, some GPs practise alternative medicine as part of their normal work, using a holistic approach. For example, they will treat hypertension or diabetes either by lifestyle changes or homeopathy first; however, if these treatments are not successful, they will then use conventional evidence-based treatment.

In Luxembourg, the use of alternative medicine is more extreme than elsewhere and is the only country where I thought it could be dangerous. Some GPs here practise alternative medicine. Some will try treating diseases with alternative medicine and if this fails will use evidence-based medicine. Other GPs have so much faith in alternative medicine that this is the only treatment they will use. The consequence is that some patients who need evidence-based medicine will be deprived of this and put at risk.

Practice Staff

Until about 1960, most GPs were either independent or practised in very small groups, but apart from the occasional secretary, they worked without staff. In the mid-sixties there was a big change, with a new charter negotiated between the British Medical Association (BMA) and the government, in which the latter paid a large part of the salary of staff and made other financial changes to encourage group practice.

As a result, many doctors work in groups of four or more, with purpose-built premises. The main change, though, is the growth of practice staff. It is normal now for a practice to have a team of receptionists and at least one secretary. The organisation of the building, doctors and staff has become so complex that there is usually a practice manager whose sole job is just that, although at first the practice manager would have doubled up as a secretary or senior receptionist.

Many of the medical jobs done by doctors have been passed safely onto nurses. These include tasks such as taking blood, syringing ears and doing dressings. As time passed, practices discovered that, when managing chronic disease, nurses could do much of the work safely and well. We will look at diabetes as an example of this. It is essential that patients with diabetes have their weight checked, blood pressure measured, feet examined and blood sent for many tests including sugar, HBA1C, cholesterol and kidney function. Not one of these tasks needs a doctor and many practices train their nurses to do this with a fixed routine known as a protocol. It is usual then for the patient to see the nurse first and then to come back a few days later to see the doctor, who can review the nurse's measurements, together with the results of the blood tests and inform the patient how he is doing and to make any necessary changes in treatment.

In British general practice, as well as there being the staff employed by the doctors, there are staff employed by the PCT and attached to the practices. Firstly, there are the district nurses, whose work is mainly to do the nursing of patients ill at home, but in some practices they also do clinics at the surgery. Then there are health visitors, whose work is with infants and their families. They monitor the baby's development, run the infant welfare clinics and make sure immunisations are done. Then there are midwives who run antenatal clinics for pregnant women, even though they would expect to have their babies in hospital. Lastly, there are a variety of counsellors, behaviour therapists and psychologists. In good times and with good PCTs, these would be expected to be attached to the practice and be part of the team. Less desirably they can work for all the doctors in one district from their own clinic so they are separate from the doctors.

One of the most interesting phenomena I witnessed going round Europe was the variation in the ancillary staff that were employed; not only with regards to the quantities but also in what they were allowed to do. In some countries the practices had almost a full set as we know it in the UK, but in others there were none.

There were almost no GPs employing secretaries, however large the group, and there were no lay practice managers in post, although in the practice I saw in Copenhagen, a person came in five hours a month to do the books.

Some countries with large group practices, such as Portugal or Finland, employed medical administrators who were GPs but did not see patients.

The number of staff employed in the various countries was roughly associated with the size of the groups. In Finland, for example, where the GPs work from large community clinics, there are many practice nurses under a head nurse. They partly do triage or sorting out emergency appointments, but also do general nursing duties as a nurse would do in the UK. This includes taking blood, giving routine injections, immunisations and the usual dressings. There were also receptionists. In Portugal and Spain, where I saw a large group practice, there are practice nurses who, with some exceptions, do a similar range of activities to those in the UK. Notable exceptions are cervical smears, which, unlike in Britain, are always done by doctors. It seems to be becoming increasingly difficult to recruit nurses in Portugal.

A more common structure was where there were small groups of two to four doctors, where they are provided by the system with nurses at the rate of one or two per doctor depending on the country. These are the doctors' only staff and they double up as receptionists. This was a common model and an example is Latvia, where the state pays for one nurse per doctor. The nurses' duties appear to be half administration, sorting out the appointment system, and half nursing, with duties similar to the UK, including taking blood and giving injections.

Sometimes the practice nursing was not done by nurses but by assistants. These appear to be receptionists trained to the level of a Health Care Assistant (HCA) in the UK. In the UK, a HCA is often a selected receptionist who has been trained to do some of the functions that are done by nurses, thus relieving pressure on the latter. Measuring weight and blood pressure and taking blood are the sort of things they do. The work of nurses and HCAs varies enormously, according to the country. Sometimes the nurses did phlebotomy (taking blood) but in Germany where, although nurses and HCAs (all did both nursing and reception) were allowed to take things out of the body such as blood, they were not allowed to put anything in, including any injections, not even vitamin B12. I was surprised that trained nurses were not allowed to give injections but this was quite common.

In all countries where nurses or HCAs did phlebotomy, they saw this as a natural part of their duties and the patients would expect to have their blood taken in the practice. In many countries childhood immunisations were given by doctors, sometimes GPs and others paediatricians, as this was what was expected and mothers would look askance if anyone else, including a nurse, did this. Similarly nurses rarely took cervical smears, these usually being done either by the GP or by primary care gynaecologists, although in Spain it was done by attached midwives.

Ear syringing was rarely done by nurses; sometimes GPs did them but often patients were referred to ENT specialists for this.

In Austria, there were no nurses but HCAs doubling up as receptionists. As well as being receptionists they did some nursing procedures such as ECGs, helped with the pathology (using the auto-analyser) and wrote the forms. However they did not take blood or syringe ears. The doctors I visited there gave all the injections themselves.

Holland, where there are no practice nurses, also has assistants who are trained, similar to HCAs in England. They do somewhere between one and three years of training and do not have university degrees. Their range of work includes, apart from recording blood pressure and ECGs, treating warts with liquid nitrogen, removing stitches and testing urine samples for infection. Ireland was an exception, where the two doctor practice I went to employed no nurses.

Twice I found practices, in Slovakia and the Czech Republic, where the nurse worked in the next room to the doctor, and the patient, on the way to the doctor would go through the nurse's room and stop for a consultation, including having a blood pressure check. It was interesting that they were able to synchronise their timing. The main object of these nurse consultations, however, was administrative, so that the attendance could be recorded for bureaucratic and therefore payment purposes.

The position of single-handed doctors varied. A common structure as seen in Poland, for example, is to have two practice nurses, although in Latvia and Estonia there is only one. Again, half of their time is spent nursing and the other half acting as receptionists, sorting out appointments etc. The nurses do the phlebotomy and can give the ordinary range of injections, such as would happen in the UK. There are no difficulties about nurses giving injections in Poland. Apart from these two nurse-come-receptionists, there is a cleaner and a book keeper. As elsewhere there was no practice manager or secretary.

The plight of single-handed doctors in some western countries seemed especially hard, although the doctors I met in Belgium, Luxembourg and France seemed content with their system. However to me, an English GP, their way of life seemed extraordinary by what we in our country have come to expect today.

The loneliest doctors I saw were in Belgium and Luxembourg. There I saw doctors with no staff at all except for a cleaner. As we saw earlier, the Belgian doctor had no staff at all. He carried a pocket computer which interacted with his desk-top computer and two mobile phones, three when he was on duty. As well as making the appointments, he has to receive the patients into his premises (his home in his case) and he has no nurses or HCAs. One doctor I saw in Luxembourg told me he had no staff, while another told me he had a sham receptionist, using an agency in the way some business people do. By this, I mean when patients phone, the call is answered by a receptionist in a bureau whose phone recognises the number and she claims to be the doctor's receptionist and takes messages for him.

The doctors in Luxembourg are proud of not having practice nurses, and are not allowed to by law. One was very defensive of this and critical of our system. He was horrified at the idea of all that nurses do in treating chronic disease such as I have described for diabetes, saying it was an interference in the relationship of doctor and patient. Although I understand his point of view, I do not agree with it. To me it is helpful having the nurse to do the mechanical tasks, where an agenda must be completed with there being very little chance for the patient to talk. This allows therefore a more relaxed consultation with the doctor, where all the issues can be discussed.

There may be an association between methods of payment and levels of staff. It seems that where the doctor is paid by item of service they are more likely to do tasks themselves and be paid in full rather than delegate them. This is not cynical greed but just the way some systems have evolved, and the doctors genuinely believe that either they can do the job better themselves, or their patients would not have confidence in any one lesser qualified. It certainly seems that they have more continuity of care.

There are no nurses in the general practices in France but this does not mean the doctors have to give the injections, apart from routine immunisations which are done by GPs or paediatricians. Nurses work from their own separate practices and the GPs refer the patients there when required. Patients are then entitled to reimbursement from the health care system. At least in the small practices there appeared to be no practice staff on site apart from the cleaner. The only receptionists, as in Luxembourg, work in an agency.

As many practices did not do paediatrics, there was often no need for health visitors, but the practice I saw in Cyprus had a weekly visiting health visitor who was responsible for the immunisation programme. In Sweden, as well as their having practice nurses and HCAs who, between them, do a similar range of work as here, there is also a full range of district nurses, who are all trained to the equivalent level of a health visitor and do many of the new baby checks.

In summary no country had as much and as great a range as that which we have come to expect here.

Certificates

When I decided as a child to become a doctor and then to go into general practice, I had the fantasy that my work was to see ill people and somehow make them better. It was a terrible shock right from the start of my career to discover that this was only a small part of the job. Many consultations are arranged for the purpose of getting a doctor's letter; for example, to the council about why the family needs a better house, to the court about why the man is unable to do jury service (he is too busy), why the driver needs a blue badge (his friends have one) and many more.

The most common of these was the doctor's certificate for work. When I first became a GP, I was obliged to provide any patient with a certificate, free of charge, even if they had been off work for only one day. After a few years, the system improved to three days and about twenty years ago in Britain it improved further so that now a certificate is required from the doctor only if the illness has lasted a week. Any shorter period has to be covered by a self-certificate provided by the employer and completed by the patient. Many employers dislike this system, being convinced that their workers are unlikely to tell the truth. Say a worker is obliged to take two days off because of an attack of diarrhoea. They like to ask him to get a doctor's certificate although they have never explained why. How is a doctor able to know the truth anymore than they are? It is not as though we go into the home to observe and count the poos.

The old system was terrible. A patient would come and see me with worrying symptoms. Examination often did not reveal anything wrong so I had to arrange a series of investigations to see what was going on. As the patient left, almost as an afterthought, they asked for a certificate and with experience I realized that that was what the consultation had been all about, and my time and anxiety had been wasted. The introduction of self-certification has been an enormous boon and saved many unnecessary consultations.

When travelling, I asked the GPs about their systems for certificates. I did not find the system of self certification for a week outside the UK. In most places, certificates for sickness were required after one to three days. Most often, even for one day, the patient had to inform the GP on the first day and attend for a certificate by the third day. The Estonian doctor told me that if she knew the patient well she would agree to issue a certificate after a phone call.

Unlike here, doctors would respond to the different requirements of employers of their patients, rather than having a national system. Many patients could be ill for three days before needing a certificate but if the firm wanted it, a certificate would be given after only one day's absence. Doctors usually seemed to take this for granted, but as many were paid for every consultation, they did not object. Nor did those in Denmark, where they are not expected to issue a certificate until the worker has been off four days, and then they can charge the employer for it. Again in Austria the need for a certificate depends on the employer and sometimes it is needed just for one day; if the patient feels too ill to come to surgery, the doctor will make a visit, comforted by knowing the system in his country, as we have seen, pays a much larger fee. However in Finland, where GPs are salaried, there has been a lot of discussion between representatives of GPs and the government about this problem, but the trade unions are strong in this country and the doctors have lost.

However, in Slovenia, if a patient attends just for a phlebotomy for an hour and a half, many patients will request a certificate for this, and sometimes will ask for a whole day, otherwise there is a risk of losing their job and the doctors give in to this. There are, it seems, therefore, many consultations purely for giving certificates. I was told that a survey found that ten to twenty percent of visits to GPs in this country were for administrative reasons only. Incidentally, hospital doctors in Slovenia, unlike in the UK, are not allowed to write certificates.

Occasionally the employer's occupational health doctor would sort it out, even visiting the employee at home. I met a private GP in Malta who, as a second job, worked for firms doing just this.

GPs do not have to give certificates in Holland. If the patient is off sick and needs any certificates, the employers use the equivalent of occupational health doctors. However, there is liaison between the GP and these doctors and the GP, if asked, will, with the consent of the patient, write any necessary notes to the occupational health doctor, explaining what is going on. They work together sometimes in guiding patients back to work again, particularly after a long time of absence. GPs can charge for this work. There are also guidelines for this co-operation.

Out-of-Hours

Nearly all countries have arrangements where patients can contact a GP when the surgery is closed. In the UK, at least up to the sixties, a GP would be on duty round the clock, although it was more usual to take turns with others, either partners or neighbouring practices. When I was a child in the forties, I remember my father, who was a GP who died relatively young, working with three other doctors, so he was on call one night and weekend in four. When I first came into practice in 1963, I did one in two with my partner but in 1967, when we amalgamated into a group practice and worked with another local practice, we improved to a one in eight.

Being on duty was the worst part of general practice. Although our contract specified we had to be available twenty four hours a day, it was possible to contract the work out to a deputising service. However, in the sixties this was thought to be a bad thing, done only by lazy, uncaring GPs. There was some justice for this view, which may seem arrogant. The deputising doctors, as they were known, in those days, although medically qualified, did not have to be trained GPs and were often training for a different speciality while needing to earn extra money. Also they had no connection with the patients or their history. Their mode of work seemed to be to prescribe an antibiotic to every patient they saw.

Therefore we did the work ourselves. For me, as I am not a good sleeper, being woken up at night was a problem as I have great difficulty in getting back to sleep, and found the next day difficult.

Although some of the night calls needed a doctor, others were trivial and I gave advice that they should come back to surgery the next day. Sometimes having done this, I lay awake, thinking I had been rash in my annoyance, had not taken a sufficient history and speculating as to what could go wrong. After about two hours, I would give up, drive down to the surgery to get the patient's address and go to their house and wake them all up with some excuse that I just happened to be passing on another call and I wanted to make sure the patient was not getting worse.

In the eighties, we surrendered the nights to the deputising service but the rest of it was still horrible. The week before my weekend on duty was a nightmare as I could not think about anything else. What made it worse was that, like most GPs, we kept our surgeries closed, so every patient that needed to see us had to have a house call. The cases we had to deal with varied from the difficult and necessary to the trivial and sometimes stupid. Many needed a doctor but could have waited until after the weekend with their coughs and colds, which had already lasted a few days. Solving difficult problems, however, often made the whole thing seem worthwhile and even exciting at times. As I was used to working in a group practice, I felt lonely working on my own at weekends, but when in difficulties, there was usually someone supportive at the local hospital.

Another problem was that because I was covering for patients that belonged to the other practice, even if I knew the roads, I did not know where the houses were. Many were not numbered and even if they were, I could not read the numbers at night, although a powerful torch could be useful. When possible, I asked the relatives to put all the lights on in every room in the front of the house and this helped sometimes. New building developments were the worst because it was not possible to park nearby, it could be hard to find the right block of flats and then the numbering system seemed quite arbitrary.

At the beginning, my wife could not always contact me when I was out visiting because many patients had no phone, so when I returned, she would greet me at the door with more requests and I would have to go straight out again, often to the district I had just left. In the seventies we acquired pagers and this improved matters, although when they sounded in a house with no phone, I had to beg the neighbour for the use of theirs, not knowing if I should offer to pay for the call. It could be embarrassing sitting on a stranger's staircase in their hall, explaining to someone else on the phone why they did not need to see me. If the pager sounded while in the car, I had to choose whether to go home first, knowing I would almost certainly have to go out again, or whether to find a call box that worked. Fortunately, in 1989, I acquired my first car phone and this did improve life. However, it was still an enormous relief when eleven o'clock came round, although tension built up in the preceding ten minutes, just as it does in injury time at a football match when Watford are winning by one goal.

Sometime during the nineties we at last got the idea, with the help of receptionists, to open the surgeries to emergencies on weekends. I had a session about six o'clock on Saturday and Sunday evenings and at noon on Sunday mornings. This meant that all patients who needed to see a doctor but were mobile could come and see me and save a house call. This reduced the amount of work a lot, but the tension only slightly.

Not surprisingly, all this angst was not confined to me but was nationwide, and the profession decided to do something about it. This led to doctors forming large groups for out-of-hours cover called co-ops. They usually covered about thirty to forty doctors and the GPs would work them in shifts. Some were staffed only by the GPs they covered; others hired deputising doctors who, by now, had to be fully trained GPs. They had staffed bases either in local hospitals or clinics where patients could be seen. I did some shifts either at the base from six o'clock to eleven o'clock or sometimes the house calls. These were no longer onerous, firstly because they had been accepted by another health professional, nurse or doctor, so I was spared the discussion, and secondly I was provided with a car and chauffeur so I did not have to navigate or park. It did not matter how many calls I had because when my shift was over, I handed what was unfinished to the night doctor, who was there for that purpose.

In 2003, GPs negotiated a new contract where they no longer had to be responsible for out-of-hours work, but the way that it is done has so far not changed very much. It is a bit of a muddle, with patients having the choice of phoning their GP, whose switchboard will direct them to the local co-op, going to the Accident and Emergency department of the nearest hospital or phoning NHS Direct, where they may get advice or be directed to one of the other services. I imagine this multiplication of services is expensive and there will be some rationalisation in the offing.

Are the changes over the years a good thing? For the quality of life for doctors the answer can only be "Yes" but for patients it is not so easy. If the illness was not serious, in the past they would have had to wait at home for the doctor to visit at an unknown time, as he would prioritise his visits on seriousness and, to a lesser extent, on geography and could not give an appointment. Now, after phoning the surgery and getting on to the co-op, an appointment at the base would be given so the patient can organize his day. For major illness, it is not always good. A patient could be suffering from a longstanding and serious condition such as terminal cancer and be seen by a doctor who does not know them or their history; I have come across some very distressing events because of this. Many GPs are aware of this problem and will give their mobile phone numbers to appropriate patients. There is of course no extra pay for this but, fortunately, doctors are still human and professionally involved. Having an aversion to incoming phone calls, I did not do this but phoned seriously ill patients once or twice on Saturdays and Sundays to see how they were doing and give advice and visit if necessary.

Now let us look at what I found in the rest of Europe. Almost everywhere in the EU, there was some form of co-op type out-of-hours service, but this statement hides enormous variations. It is best to divide out-of-hours into days, weekends and nights.

Sometimes the services are the responsibility of the state, which is similar to British national health practices, which have opted out of out-of-hours care. They usually use some sort of triage system that will know when to send a GP. In a few countries, the triage person is able to differentiate between general practice and secondary care. Thus if, say, a patient phoned with acute abdominal pain, arrangements would be made for them to see a surgeon direct without troubling a GP.

However, in some countries the doctors have to pay for the out-of-hours service. In Poland, for example, evenings and weekends are done entirely by an emergency service and the GP has to pay a subscription to this service out of his capitation fees. The subscription is fixed depending on the number of patients at risk. The amount of times the patients use the service is irrelevant to the cost. The patients will either come up to the centre or be visited by a chauffeur-driven car.

It appears to be a paradox to call day service 'out-of-hours', but when doctors have finished their work for the day, someone must look after their patients. In Poland, for example, at least one doctor in a group practice must stay on duty until the co-op service starts and, as we will see, the trainee may be left to mind the shop with suitable telephone cover. If he is away, or if there is no trainee, the practice nurse will cover. In Denmark, for example, the doctor told me that she and her partners often all finish by 2.30pm and want to go home, and persuade a neighbouring doctor to cover for them until the first co-op type shift starts at 4pm. In Sweden, as we have noted, visit requests coming in during the day are left, if possible, for the emergency service when it comes on at 5pm.

In most countries the weekends mean all day Saturday and Sunday but occasionally, for example in Lithuania, Saturday morning counts as a weekday. A common arrangement is for the local GPs to run a co-op, doing the work themselves, although they usually have the choice of opting out, paying or persuading a colleague or even a locum to do the work for them. If they cannot get a substitute or if they are let down they must do the duty themselves. Some countries have rules, however, that all GPs must do a minimum number of out-of-hours sessions themselves to remain on the register. Again, in some places doctors have to do a minimum of nights on call to remain on the register but everywhere I found this, doctors were excused this requirement if they were older than fifty four. There is no such obligation in Britain.

The practice I visited in Germany was in East Berlin, where there are too many GPs so there is no difficulty in running primary care services at nights and weekends, which is done by the equivalent of co-ops. Any doctor can volunteer to do night work and weekend work and plenty do because they need to earn extra money. The work at night is done entirely by house-calls, patients are not seen at any centre and the doctors are provided with a chauffeur-driven car.

In Slovenia, all the GPs in town have to take their turn to work weekends and they do either a Saturday or Sunday and do two of these days a month for twenty-four hours. Even if these twenty-four hours are a Sunday, they are expected to come back to work on the Monday and work in the normal way. However, they do accumulate spare hours by doing these weekends and eventually after a few weekends they can take a day off which, of course, has to be paid for by the partners doing double work. (The doctor actually said "sweat blood" as locums are rarely employed in her practice.) They do not have to do weekday evenings which are covered from a central facility.

The Finnish system is similar but voluntary. After four o'clock on a weekday, work ends. One doctor has to be on duty until ten o'clock at night and stays in the centre. On Saturday and Sunday during the day, also, the GPs have to take it in turns to be on duty until ten o'clock at night. They are paid a lot extra for this and so enough of them volunteer to do it. It is usually done by a rota, involving their doing it two or three times a month. If there are not sufficient volunteers, the medical administrator of the centre will have to allocate doctors to take their turn. During the night in the town, from ten o'clock until morning, out-of-hours calls are dealt with by GPs from one centre, involving the whole town. Any GP can volunteer to do this and indeed one of the GPs from the community centre I visited does; he chooses Friday or Saturday night, so he is fit to do his weekday work afterwards.

In Lisbon, the very large health centre I saw is open for emergencies until 10pm in the evenings and on Saturdays, and the doctors have to take turns to staff the health centre at these times, when there will be two to three doctors present. During the night and on Sundays, patients are seen in emergency clinics at hospitals. These clinics are run by GPs and any GP is able to take on this work and is very highly paid to do this.

Sometimes there is no co-op of GPs but the state system or the health insurance society equivalent provides the out-of-hours service. It is not always clear who these doctors are or if they are vocationally trained for general practice. (Vocational training is the British term for training for general practice.) In Spain these doctors come into the health centre and take over. In Italy, again, the doctors covering out-of-hours have not been vocationally trained or necessarily done general practice. The service starts at 8pm and is run from hospitals. Mostly, nights are similar to evenings and weekends.

In some countries, there was no primary care out-of-hours service provided by the state system. Patients had a choice of A&E, calling an ambulance or contacting a private GP. I was told in Sweden this was because general practice at night had not been found to be cost-effective.

In Cyprus this absence of primary care started at 2.30pm on weekdays, when the GPs' work finishes. After this time patients must choose to wait until the next working day or, if they cannot, they again have the choice of A&E, calling an ambulance or a private doctor. On Saturday afternoons, all day Sundays and evenings, the same system operates in Lithuania.

In Greece, in rural health areas, patients would go to the health centre during the night or on weekends, and there would be some administrator there who would wake up the appropriate doctor, such as the internist or the paediatrician. As we saw earlier, the rural health centres have satellite centres in villages, staffed by a doctor on his own in training. He is responsible for the patients on his patch round the clock. In the towns, the clinics (which are run by various unions) are closed at nights and on weekends, and patients are expected to go to the A&E department, where they are treated.

The arrangements in France are similar to many countries in that doctors have to provide a twenty-four hour service, but they can use emergency services at night and weekends, especially in

Paris, although outside Paris they have to take their turn in a rota unless they can pay someone else to do it.

Paris has, I believe, a unique system in that the service is staffed by trained GPs who do not have their own surgeries. They will leave a scribbled note for the regular GP. These doctors are not locums but working out-of-hours at no fixed address, so to speak, is their career. It seems, therefore, that there are two groups of GPs, one of which is the day group, with their own surgery and practice and the other, an out-of-hours group with no premises. Both are paid item of service fees by the patient, who is largely reimbursed by the authorities.

In Latvia, as in the UK, some doctors give selected patients their mobile phone numbers. This may happen in other countries (see Estonia below) but I was not told of any others.

The practice I visited in Estonia is unusual in that all patients are given the doctors' mobile telephone numbers. In the waiting room, I was impressed to see a list of the doctors' names, the hours when they do their sessions and their mobile telephone numbers. I was told by the GP I interviewed that although her mobile phone often rings in the evening she will give advice but if a patient needs to be visited, and this is some way off from where she is at that moment, she will advise them to ring the emergency service to ask for a doctor to visit or to take themselves to an emergency department. She very rarely gets telephoned at night.

It seems that where doctors are single-handed, such as in Belgium, although there is a state-run emergency service, the doctor is likely to remain available himself because it is only by seeing patients that he will earn a living.

Malta is different from all this. General practice seems to be in a permanent state of 'in hours'. Doctors seem to be in groups of twenty five, working in shifts of five doctors at a time, and these shifts run continuously throughout the night and weekend, so in theory there is no emergency service, just a normal service around the clock. However, doctors still get annoyed if a patient turns up for a routine matter like a blood pressure check during the night and may refuse to do it.

Complaints and Litigation

The NHS has always had a built-in complaints system. Up until the eighties, if a patient felt they had had poor, rude or incompetent service they could complain to the predecessor of the PCT. The complaint would be considered by a service committee who could fix a hearing in front of a panel, which was a mixture of lay people and GPs. If found guilty, the doctor could be reprimanded or, if the case were bad, they could be fined by having a chunk of their earnings withheld. The whole process took months and completely dominated the doctor's life, even if he thought the complaint malicious or trivial. The procedure was highly confrontational, usually leading to a complete and permanent rupture of any relationship with the patient and the removal of him and his family from the practice.

Fortunately the process has been replaced by an 'in-house' system. Each practice has to have some system in place and mostly they are similar. In my practice, the practice manager is the designated complaints officer. He deals with administrative complaints. Medical complaints are dealt with by one of the partners to whom the practice manager passes them. I was the medical complaints officer for my practice, so I dealt with medical complaints unless they were directed at me, in which case another partner handled them.

It seems to work well. Although the complaints are few, they are satisfying to deal with. If I think the patient's complaint is due to a misunderstanding, after reading it carefully and questioning the doctor to whom it refers, I send back a detailed letter explaining what happened. If the patient is not satisfied, I invite him to come, with a friend or officer of the PCT if he likes, to a meeting where we discuss the whole thing. The meetings take about an hour and at the end of it, both sides are usually satisfied, are in agreement and the relationship continues often warmer than before. If it appears the doctor is at fault, I arrange the meeting anyway and again the events are reviewed and the doctor will be able to explain what happened and apologize. This is nearly always what the patient wanted and again there is a happy outcome. Later the practice will review what occurred and see if lessons can be learnt from it to avoid it happening again.

For me, after the changes in out-of-hours arrangements, this is the greatest improvement for the quality of life for GPs since I have been in practice. Complaints changed from a threat hanging over one to a learning experience.

Apart from complaints, there is the risk of litigation and the defence arrangements that doctors make. I have not personally been sued but I have seen the occasional case in my practice, although none have been successful. However, in England, as in the USA, a successful complaint can lead to enormous damages, which seem to be increasing all the time. Therefore doctors belong to defence organizations, the two best known being the Medical Protection Society (MPS) and the Medical Defence Union (MDU). Probably all practising doctors in the UK are members of some defence body; indeed, I remember that my father was. In many jobs, such membership is compulsory, including working as a GP in the NHS. Related to the increase of damages awarded, the subscriptions have grown fast; for a full-time GP they are currently about four and a half thousand pounds a year.

European doctors outside the UK do not expect to be sued and take it for granted that their patients trust them. When I asked about it, doctors were usually taken aback and gave the impression they did not think this an important subject. More than one said that they assumed the problem would eventually loom larger and one day they would be like the United States in this respect. They never said "like the United Kingdom", obviously not realising that defensive medicine in our country was more like that in the United States than continental Europe. Similarly, it seemed that formal complaints were as rare as litigation. The amount of litigation is increasing, I was told, in Holland.

In the Czech Republic, the GPs belong to a chamber which is a mixture of defence organisation, union and ethical body, and membership is compulsory. This will defend them against complaints, providing they have done the minimum of keeping up to date required by the Czech authorities. In other countries, the doctors pay for insurance but it is usually only a modest amount; for instance, in Denmark it is about a hundred euros a year and in Spain last year it was a hundred and sixty four euros. In Sweden, their medical association provides free legal representation but, although most doctors are members, it is not a requirement of practice. In Denmark, membership of the medical association which provides defence was compulsory until the end of 2006 but is now voluntary. I did not raise this topic sufficiently often to know how widespread, if at all, having defence insurance is a requirement to be a general practitioner, as it is in the UK.

I must say something about chaperones. When I was training in hospital, a male doctor would make sure a nurse was present if he were to do any breast or intimate examination of a woman. I found that this was not the case in general practice, even though the MPS advised doctors that they should always have a chaperone. Until about five years ago, it was never on the agenda. I and my colleagues just examined patients when necessary. In the days before we had staff, a single-handed doctor could be alone in a building with his patient. Also, on house-calls, the doctor and the patient could be the only people present. Obviously, in theory, this put the woman at risk of assault and the doctor at risk of false accusations. I never personally heard of a case but occasionally read of one in the press. In the last few years, there has been so much extra pressure to have chaperones that an increasing number of doctors do now.

My practice took advice from the respective defence bodies

who were adamant that doctors must offer a chaperone for each examination. Sitting in the room is not enough; she must be behind the curtain, sitting at the head end of the couch to protect the woman's privacy. Because of the nature of what was going on, the chaperone ought to be another health professional, such as a female partner or nurse. Unfortunately, we do not have spare doctors or nurses sitting about so this was not practicable. We have compromised and invite a receptionist in who sits outside the curtain and so far this seems to have worked.

On my journey I asked male doctors if they required chaperones. They were all even more surprised at this question than they were about the ones on being sued, and appeared not to have thought of the problem. One male doctor is also a school doctor and sees school pupils up to the age of twenty on their own, although there is a nurse in a room outside. Even the GPs who had no staff and could be alone in the premises, and sometimes these were in their homes, did not see it as a problem and took it for granted that patients and doctors trusted each other.

It is difficult to understand why we are so different from the rest of the EU in terms of trust. I understand that in the old communist parts of Europe, patients may have had difficulty complaining and may not have had easy access to lawyers but in the countries of Western Europe the culture is more similar to the East than here. I know that, like the United States, we are a litigious society but this does not explain it all. For example, the change in need for chaperones seems to have grown out of nowhere in the last few years. One thought that I will discuss later is that the break down of continuity of care, which is happening so rapidly in England, has fractured the doctor-patient relationship, preventing the doctor being seen as the patient's friend.

Continuing Medical Education and Related Topics

Although doctors, being professional, have to keep up-to-date, the arrangements vary, as do the requirements for this by each state. In the UK, since I have been in practice, there have been many changes. At present every doctor in all specialities is expected each year to make a personal learning plan (PLP) for themselves and document it each time in a portfolio. Although there is no supervision for this at present, each doctor must have an appraisal annually by a colleague; the system being known as peer appraisal. In general practice, GPs volunteer and, if suitable, are selected and trained for this task. The portfolio is submitted about two weeks in advance and the appraiser and appraisee meet for two to three hours and study it together. The appraiser will congratulate the appraisee on work done, review the past year and may suggest some new areas to study and help to devise the PLP for the coming year. The PLP will highlight areas where the doctor feels he is weak or sometimes subjects he wants to concentrate on so that he can provide a special and excellent service for the whole practice, such as running the diabetic clinic. The learning needs can be met any way the doctor chooses. He may study topics on the internet, learn from a hospital consultant or go on courses. If he goes to lectures, he will be expected but not forced to have made some reflections on what has been learnt and these will be in the portfolio. He may organize some of his learning in the regular educational meetings that occur in-house in many practices.

Another aspect of keeping up-to-date is Significant Event Analysis. If anything in the doctor's professional life has gone wrong, from an unexpected death to a reasonable complaint, the doctor will discuss this with his practice in a meeting and they will study what went wrong in a non-judgmental way and see what steps could be taken to prevent a recurrence. There will be a later follow up to ensure that all in the practice are observing any new procedures adopted. The doctor will put the minutes of the discussion in his portfolio. The NHS takes this form of learning so seriously that they award points for it, so these discussions are in the doctors' financial interests as well as fulfilling a professional need.

In most countries there is some form of reaccreditation. This means doctors no longer have the right when qualified to assume they can be doctors for life just by passing their exams; they must demonstrate that they are still studying and do not get behind. In the UK at present, reaccreditation does not occur but it is being developed. It is thought that the system will be to award reaccreditation after five successful appraisals. There has been some discussion that for this to be successful the appraisers would have more supervisory powers and may demand evidence of good work.

Continuing Medical Education (CME) is important in most countries and is the most common, and usually only, route to reaccreditation. Doctors are expected to take part in approved learning experiences. These could be lectures, of a bums-on-seats variety, where the participant could sleep through much of them with no reflection afterwards, conferences or distance-learning through journals and the internet. Occasionally, there were in house clinical meetings, but significant event discussions were rare and some doctors have not heard of the concept. They do occur in the large practices in Slovenia with both the partners and trainees attending and they seem to be well-run.

Doctors told me in a few countries that they belong to study groups outside their practice. They may be run on Balint lines but seem to be more informal. (Michael Balint was a psychoanalyst who held seminars for GPs in the fifties in the Tavistock Clinic in North London. Doctors studied their feelings towards their patients, leading to a better understanding of how to make the doctor-patient relationship work to help solve the patients' problems. These groups are still used today, often as part of training for general practice. To many of us, Balint is known as a father of general practice.) They can be used to discuss significant events but again informally. My Belgian host told me that although he was single-handed, he belonged to a local group of fourteen doctors who met at his house four times a year to discuss clinical subjects.

The amount of study that is done is measured in hours or points depending on the system. Often there is a minimum required for the equivalent of reaccreditation, although the sanctions imposed, if at all, when this is not achieved are not the same everywhere. Often the doctor could be suspended if the total is not reached, although in Slovenia a warning is given six months before and I am told this almost always makes the doctor take action so suspension is avoided. In Italy, the sanction is GPs are not allowed to register new patients until they do the necessary CME. In Malta, rather than sanctions, doctors need to do about nine hours work of CME to be eligible to become members of their college.

In Hungary, there is a similar sort of scheme with doctors having to acquire a minimum number of points over a five year period by attending various educational events including lectures and workshops. If they do not accumulate enough points, they are removed from the register and not allowed to see patients until they have remedied this. After the first five years of this plan, there was an amnesty, but the next review period is in 2009, when doctors will actually be struck off if they haven't reached the required total.

In Slovakia, if the doctors do not acquire sufficient points in five years, they are forced to take an examination and, if they fail, they are removed from the register. As far as is known this has never happened.

As we saw in the previous chapter, in the Czech Republic the Chamber will not defend doctors who have not done sufficient CME. In Germany the sanction for not acquiring enough points is a reduction of pay for doctors by the health insurance agency, while in Belgium it is a reduction of reimbursement for their patients; naturally these patients ask embarrassing questions.

The Dutch sanction, if they do not achieve their forty hours' CME in five years, is for them to get a very severe warning and then get one year's grace and have to do far more hours than would have been necessary otherwise. If this is not achieved, they would be removed from the register, but probably doctors do not get to this stage.

In Lithuania, as well as needing enough CME points for doctors to stay on the register, it is a requirement that all doctors work for at least three years in any five.

Some countries, such as Finland, France and Poland, have no sanctions at all and it is almost the same in Austria, where enough CME points need to be obtained each year to get a certificate; however, it does not seem to matter if this is not obtained. These countries therefore seem to have no equivalent of reaccreditation in place.

In Greece, newly-qualified doctors need to have some form of points and there are three or four educational events in the big towns each year where most doctors go, and the younger doctors queue up afterwards for certificates. They need these points to graduate from houseman (newly-qualified hospital doctor) eventually to a fully-qualified specialist. Once they are fully-qualified specialists they may go to these events but there is no compulsion that they should do so. Thus here again, there seems to be no form of reaccreditation for established doctors.

In summary, where CME is linked to accreditation, there is an ingenious variety of sanctions which tend to be lightly used.

These systems for reaccreditation do not apply in the UK, Ireland, Sweden and Denmark. In Denmark, GPs are paid when they are on courses and they notify the health authority when they do this; that is the only means by which the health authority knows who has any continuing medical education, but there are no sanctions if it is not done.

With the partial exception of Holland, mentioned below, requiring a minimum of CME was the only method I found of reaccreditation.

The absence of reaccreditation does not mean, therefore, there is no CME; far from it. It is just that, as no evidence of further study is required for doctors to stay on the register, some slip through the net. For example, the Irish doctor I saw arranges his personal development plan, which is voluntary, through the Irish College of General Practitioners. In Portugal, there is no reaccreditation, no personal development plans and no significant event discussions, but the health centre I visited did arrange in-house clinical meetings with outside speakers. Health centres provide in-house clinical meetings but attendance at these varies and is poor or non-existent in the practice I attended.

In Sweden, there is no requirement by the state that the doctors should have continuing medical education, but many do. The GP I visited belongs to a group of dedicated doctors outside her practice, who meet on alternate Monday evenings to discuss various subjects in a group. This way they keep up to date. There are also regular practice meetings: these are held weekly, some being administrative and some clinical. Locally, the county primary care board arranges courses and CME days for its GPs regularly, and one of the GPs in the district is employed part time to arrange these events. Nationally, many GPs take part in the annual meetings of the Swedish Society of Medicine, and the Swedish Association of General Practice (sister organization to the The Royal College of General Practitioners).

CME in Luxembourg is entirely voluntary. The doctors tell me it is in their interest not to get out of date and they read journals and go to meetings, and one of the doctors I saw studies in a group. There is, however, no requirement for continuing medical education and there are no plans for reaccreditation. In a country in which freedom from controls for both doctors and patients is almost an obsession and they are very proud of their independence. I am told that they will not be forced into doing anything.

Study leave for CME is variable. For salaried doctors or those on capitation fees, sometimes it is paid; in Portugal the GPs have fifteen paid days for study leave but what they do during this time is not monitored. In Spain there is a week's study leave each year but again there is no check on how this time is used. In Malta, doctors have to apply for study leave, the granting of which is not automatic.

Slovene doctors are permitted eleven study days a year but as the practice I visited did not employ locums, and I had the impression that the absence of locums was widespread, the remaining partners had to undertake a bigger workload.

For others, however, it has to come out of holiday time. Doctors on item-of-service payments would find it expensive to take study leave during surgery hours. I did though meet some WONCA doctors who were single-handed and were prepared to go to a conference in Florence.

In the EU, outside the UK there is no peer appraisal; the only appraisals I came across were in Austria, Finland, Slovenia and, rather vaguely, in Cyprus. In Austria, an annual questionnaire (to evaluate the quality of the practice, there are prescribed standards which must be fulfilled) is sent to the doctor asking him about the management of his patients (How is the practice reachable for the disabled? How are appointments made? What kind of instruments and medical devices does he have? How are medical records stored and managed? etc.). If an appraiser of the quality control system, which is supervised by the ministry of health, is not satisfied with the answers or if there have been complaints, he will then make an educational visit to the GP where they will discuss the work together, and this will act as some form of appraisal. In this appraisal, sanctions are possible.

In Finland, every doctor in the community health centre is appraised annually by the Deputy Chief Physician, in a meeting of about an hour. This meeting may discuss the doctor's usual work, but there are no personal development plans implemented. All employees in the centre are also appraised by their own managers. Appraisal is expected in Slovenia but this will be by faculty doctors rather than peers. In Cyprus, a doctor in the local authority writes an annual report of every GP. They don't necessarily interview every GP annually, but the report will say how they get on with colleagues, staff and patients. The GP told me she did not know how they obtain this information.

In Holland during the last year there has been a scheme where a practice can apply for what they call accreditation (proof or acknowledgement of quality) when it meets certain criteria for quality. It takes three years to fulfill the procedure and get this accreditation. More than five hundred and twenty practices (1.2 million patients) are already in.

Almost every doctor I met seemed surprised at the notion of peer appraisal and told me he knew of no plans for it to come in his country.

The issue of poorly-performing doctors is important in this country. This was highlighted after the Bristol tragedy, when children having heart surgery were dying in greater numbers than expected and, on inquiry, it was found that two of the surgeons were not properly trained for the work that they were doing and the hospital administrator, a doctor, had known about it and taken no action. One of the surgeons and the hospital administrator were struck off the register. The Shipman case was really irrelevant as he was a murderous villain rather than incompetent. Since the Bristol case the General Medical Council (GMC) has made it absolutely clear that if any doctor knows of a colleague who is under-performing, no matter what the cause, and does not take action, and this leads to harm to patients, he will be considered to be guilty of unprofessional behavior and liable to be struck off himself.

Outside Britain there were no arrangements for identifying or dealing with poorly-performing doctors. When I asked GPs about this they were always taken aback and rather uncomfortable. Usually they appeared not to have come across the issue. When pressed, they would say that they would speak to the doctor in question and it was clear that, firstly, they were more concerned for the doctor than the patients and, more importantly, it was not their problem. This was not callousness, it was just that they had rarely had to consider this, and following a discussion they agreed that patients must be protected.

I was told that Irish doctors have a duty to patients if there are poorly-performing doctors, but there are no established systems in place that are known. This seems to be the crux, in that even if doctors are concerned about poorly-performing colleagues, they have no established systems in which to take action.

The matter is rather different in Finland because GPs work in large groups managed by doctors. Here, complaints would go to the medical administrator who is responsible. The one I met was in the middle of dealing with such a problem, causing her great anxiety.

It is thought that in Holland the way of dealing with poorly-performing doctors and the seriousness of it is moving towards the UK's ideas of this.

Training For General Practice

There is supposed to be an EU regulation that, throughout the region, doctors must undergo specialist training for general practice and pass some sort of test of competence, known as a Summative Assessment, before they can do any unsupervised work in general practice. Because of this, a doctor cannot even be a locum in this country without the required period of training and a document called a Vocational Training Certificate (or an equivalent) to prove he has acquired competence.

As expected, training for general practice varies, but before describing my findings abroad, I will give a brief summary of what is required in this country. As in the rest of Europe, our system is always undergoing rapid change, but I will set out the general principles. For many years, GPs in training were reasonably enough called trainees, but about ten years ago the name was changed to registrars. It has reverted this season to trainee again. I will use either term and I intend them to have the same meaning.

After graduation, all doctors, regardless of the speciality they will choose (and please remember that general practice is considered a speciality in this and many other countries), must undergo two years of Foundation School training, which are usually spent as six attachments of four months each in different hospital specialities. In the second year, fifty-five percent of doctors are attached to general practice for four months.

211

Since August 2007, the General Medical Council (GMC), the regulatory body of British medicine, registers only EU GPs who have done a minimum of five years postgraduate training i.e. two foundation years and three for their speciality.

After this period, the doctor chooses his speciality and, if he selects general practice, he undergoes a period of GP specialist training. The training is done in GP Specialist Training Schemes, which take place in groups centred on main hospitals. This training period lasts three years, and half to two thirds of this time is spent working in various hospital departments, often for six months at a time. The GP specialist trainee chooses the specialities that are most relevant to his future in general practice. These include a selection of paediatrics, obstetrics and gynaecology, care of the elderly, A&E and psychiatry. The rest of the time is spent in general practice. He is taught by a GP, called a trainer in the UK. Trainers are selected for their qualities as doctors and teachers and also the quality of the practice in which they work. As part of the selection process, each practice is visited at the outset and at regular intervals of not more than three years. The trainers in each scheme are obliged to join a workshop, which meets about three times a term. Trainers, as well as being paid, benefit in kind in that, as the registrars progress during their training, they are able to do a significant part of the work of the practice. However, they would not normally be left on their own without the trainer or a partner on the premises.

During the whole of the three years, all the doctors learning on the scheme are expected to join a study group weekly in term time. These groups are usually held in the hospital. An important component of training in the UK is study of consultation techniques. This is done in several ways but a key one is for the registrar to make a video tape of the live consultation. This is done only after the patient has given informed and personal consent and no picture is taken of the physical examination.

At the end of the training period, the registrars must demonstrate their competence and this is done by passing an examination to become a member of the Royal College of General

Practitioners (RCGP). Only when this is achieved is the doctor allowed to enter general practice as a locum, assistant or partner. A partner, by the way, is the doctor you know most and your doctor is likely to be one and have his name on the list on the front door. The locums and assistants are employees of the partners. It is incidentally not common to find any GPs, except when doing out-of-hours work, in the rest of Europe who are not the equivalent of partners.

Now let us see how all this compares with training on the continent. Throughout most of the EU there is vocational training for general practice and although there are often similarities to the UK system, the variations are enormous. It must be remembered that, as in our country, almost everywhere else it is evolving all the time. It is usually, however loosely, similar to vocational training for general practice in Britain in that there is usually a hospital component and a general practice component, sometimes with both being worked simultaneously. The length of schemes varies and can last up to five years.

I was surprised to find that in a couple of places there seemed to be no training and, even where there was, there was sometimes no compulsory assessment at the end.

I will briefly deal with the exceptions, then discuss the hospital component, followed by the general practice part, and then we will look at the trainers. Finally there will be descriptions of Summative Assessment. More than in previous sections in this work, I shall have to keep referring to individual countries because so many of them at present have unique systems for the various components of training.

In Italy at present there is no vocational training as we know it. When doctors qualify, they must do a month in general practice and then two months in hospital and then they are free to enter general practice as a principal and build up their list. There is some variation throughout the country. Apparently there are the universities, who do not encourage vocational training and do not agree with the syndicates, which are large groups of general practitioners who are hoping to bring in a three year vocational training scheme.

There is no vocational training in Malta and it is possible to go straight from medical school into general practice. However, their academic college of general practice, the equivalent of our RCGP, is hoping to arrange for vocational training, which will be a course of three years, half of which will be spent in general practice, and trainers will be trained by a 'Training for Trainers' course. Although, at first, vocational training will be voluntary, it is thought that it will eventually be harder for doctors to get good jobs without this training.

The hospital part varies between countries. In many countries there is an emphasis on internal medicine, where much more time is spent working in this speciality than any other hospital one. A popular scheme is to concentrate on internal medicine, even for up to eighteen months, followed by short periods for other specialities, usually of four months. Sometimes trainee GPs are expected to do paediatric and gynaecology posts even though they work in countries where these disciplines are practised by primary care paediatricians and gynaecologists, instead of general practitioners. Often there are quick rotations through other specialties, such as Ear Nose and Throat surgery (ENT) or orthopaedics, lasting only a few weeks each, rather like being a medical student. An example of this would be Cyprus, where six months is spent on internal medicine in the hospital. Added to this, there is a selection of six months in surgery, four months' paediatrics, four months' psychiatry, three months' gynaecology, three months' cardiology, two months' ophthalmology, two months' dermatology, two months at the X-ray department, one month's epidemiology in a university in Greece, seven months in Outpatients, one month endocrinology, one month neurology, one month at the chest clinic, and three months at the casualty department of the general hospital. This is followed by four months in primary care under the supervision of a GP. At the end of the training the doctors have examinations at the Greece University.

The length of vocational training varies; in Hungary and Sweden, for example, it lasts for five years. In the former, for the first twenty-seven months the doctors do a variety of modules, working in the hospital, although throughout they have a GP mentor. After this, they take a licentiate examination in family medicine and then can work as a GP, but they are paid the basic rate. At the end of five years, they take an examination in family medicine and, if they pass this, are fully-fledged general practitioners and are paid an additional twenty percent. During this period, they have a trainer whom they see once a week, except towards the end. The trainer will sometimes sit in with them. In Sweden ,two years of the time are spent in general practice, the rest in hospital, the longest post there being internal medicine which lasts six to twelve months, and the other hospital jobs are of four months duration. The training in general practice lasts from two months to two years; in the latter instance, it is usually broken up.

In Holland, two of the three years of the scheme are done in general practice, being split in half with the hospital component sandwiched in the intervening year. It consists of a rotation of three or four months each, out of a choice of the relevant major specialties with, psychiatry and being a doctor in a nursing home being mandatory.

In Slovenia, where the vocational training lasts four years, general practice is done through much of this time on one day a week. These days alternate between going to the trainer's practice and working with the trainer, and the trainer going to their practice and teaching them there. In the first part of the training they sit in with the trainer, then the trainer sits in with them and then they work on their own. In much of this time, the doctors will attend some form of day-release, usually in their university hospitals.

In no country was the trainer selected by a practice visit.

The trainers in Slovenia are selected and trained but are paid modestly. In Latvia, before Perestroika, trainers were trained and sent on courses in Moscow or Kiev for training, but this is no longer thought to be necessary.

In Austria and the Czech Republic, vocational training has been affected by a shortage of funds to pay trainers or trainees. In Austria, the position is fluid in that, although vocational training consists of a three year rotation going round hospital departments for short periods, there used to be a six month general practice component. This, however, had to be abandoned as there was never enough money to pay a reasonable number of trainees. A group of doctors aligned to WONCA are hoping to get an addition to the current vocational training of six months; sitting in with GPs. Also in the future, they plan to have a specialist course for general practice with a curriculum of six years, eighteen months' working with a GP included. In the Czech Republic, where vocational training is five years, doctors are attached to a trained trainer for the second half. They should be paid, but at present there is money for only fifty trainees, while two hundred and fifty are coming through the system. This, I was told, is a major unresolved national crisis. There are problems in Slovakia, where vocational training lasts five years but during this time, the trainees are not paid, and therefore very few apply for the scheme. There is a big shortage of young GPs there and the average age of the GPs in this country is about fifty-four.

In many places, trainers are not paid, the idea being that any work done by the trainee compensates for the effort put in by the trainer. Although this is the position in Spain, there is a surplus of trainers there, so no trainer can train for long. These trainers are selected but not trained. In Sweden, which has an advanced system of vocational training, although the trainers are not paid, their clinic is, so they are free to spend time on training.

Poland has a compulsory and well-thought out vocational training system. The first few months of this are done in general practice and then there is a hospital rotation, including internal medicine, paediatrics and geriatrics, the length of posts varying. Doctors are paid during this time. If the trainees have done internal medicine before their vocational training, the course is shortened. After the hospital work, they do another one and a half years in general practice with a selected and trained trainer. The trainer is called a master and the trainee an intern. The master is responsible for the intern in all three phases of the vocational training. That is, the general practice before the hospital work, the hospital work and the last one and a half years. During this last period, he gives two tutorials a week, one of which will be discussing topics and the other, patients. Rather than receiving money for being a master, he is paid in kind as the intern can look after his patients, giving him

216

a chance to leave the surgery. He leaves the interns only when he thinks they are safe. At the end of vocational training, they have to pass state specialty exams, which are quite difficult.

In some places trainees were not allowed to do visits on their own and although they could in Lithuania, they must not prescribe for the patient until they have discussed the case with the trainer. In some countries, when they see patients in the surgery they can not write prescriptions themselves. In others, such as we have seen in Poland, they have more responsibility even, sometimes being left in charge of the surgery if the trainer is out at a meeting.

In Holland, trainees video their consultations and take them to their day-release course; apart from that, I did not come across any place in Europe where video-recording was used in the consultation, and I visited quite a few academic practices. Where the consultation was studied, such as in Hungary, this would have been at the day-release, using actors or peers for role play, apart from case discussion by some trainers.

Denmark has a system with some similarities to ours, in which all doctors, including those who do not intend to be GPs, must do six months of general practice training during their eighteen months of pre-registration. If they think they might want to do general practice, they then do another six months of general practice and then if, after that they decide they want to become GPs, they do a three year course of vocational training, two years spent rotating round hospital specialties, as in the UK, but before this there is another six months based in general practice and at the end, a final six months based in the same practice. The practice that I visited which had one full time partner and two part-time ones, always has two trainees, the one working together with the part-time doctors might be the new trainee and the other with the full time doctor the old one, or the other way round. Trainers are paid to have the trainees during the first six-month period because these doctors cannot contribute much work, but the trainers themselves have to pay part of the salary to the second, more experienced trainee, in return for which the trainee does a significant amount of work. The trainers go through most cases in every surgery of the junior trainee, but not nearly so often for the senior one. They are expected to spend half an hour a day with the trainees. The trainers are selected and have at the beginning a week's training course, but then nothing further; as usual, outside the UK, there are no trainers' workshops. At the completion of vocational training, trainees have a summative assessment with many different things tested by the university. It is not clear how consultation technique is tested because it is not normal for them to video their consultations in their training practice.

France has a unique system of training for general practice and I am afraid it is rather sad. Shortly after the medical students qualify as doctors, they take a big examination which is competitive, in that the results are ranked. The top doctors get the first choice of careers and they mostly choose to become specialists in hospitals. General practice is not nearly so popular, because it is much lower paid and, although unfairly, has a lower status. Morale in French general practice is not good. However, once the doctors enter general practice, since 2004 they have had training which is similar to ours. Added to this, uniquely in France, during their whole three years, trainees have to prepare their portfolio and they have quite a vigorous assessment. They are also required to write an essay of twenty to thirty pages, for example, about a particularly difficult case and all the issues they have learnt from that. To get a diploma in medicine all students have also to write a thesis.

As can be imagined, summative assessment, where in place, takes different forms. Trainees' portfolios were popular, as were Objective Structured Clinical Examinations (OSCEs). OSCEs are an examination where there is a room or area with several stations. The candidate goes to each one in turn, and is confronted by a problem which he must solve. He could be asked to interpret an ECG, comment on a case history or explain abnormal blood tests, but the examples seem infinite. Sometimes, as in Poland, there is a stringent state speciality examination and sometimes a combination of methods.

In Holland, summative assessment consists partly of the trainer's report, which is very comprehensive, as the trainer has spent the whole of the third year with the trainee preparing for this, and also portfolio work done throughout the three years, which has to satisfy the course organiser before the doctor gets his vocational training certificate.

In Sweden where, as we have seen, vocational training is for five years, there is a choice of summative assessment. On application to the National Board of Health and Welfare for specialist status, the head of the practice, the trainer and the vocational training counsellor together certify that the doctor has achieved the goals of the curriculum. There is also a specialist examination in general practice at the end of the five years, which only about fifteen percent of doctors sit at present and there are no sanctions for the rest; however, a modular summative assessment programme is being developed.

As in many other aspects of general practice, the system in Finland is different from anywhere else. After doctors qualify, they have a choice of two years' or six years' vocational training. For the two year course, they do six months in hospital, nine months' primary care and nine months in either one or the other. There is no summative assessment at the end of these two years. However, if they choose to be specialists in general practice, they have six years of vocational training with a difficult examination at the end. This involves two years working in hospital and four years working in general practice, not necessarily in the same one. The GP trainers are selected and trained but not paid for this. There seems to be no discrimination by patients or managers between the briefly-trained GPs and the fully-trained GP specialists.

In summary, the main difference in vocational training between the UK and continental Europe is the lack of training of trainers and anything like trainers' workshops. Trainers are not always paid. Except for Holland, live consultations are not studied on videotape. Summative assessment is sometimes absent or optional.

The common similarities are having components of hospital rotations, general practice work and hospital or university release.

Comparisons

By the time I had seen my last doctor, I had noticed several themes which I would like to look at briefly. Although I was left feeling much more positive about the British NHS than before I started, there were some points of practice on the continent which are certainly worth considering. It is not surprising that, after the examination of twenty-four foreign systems, I could find areas where we might want to consider change. I would like to look at the issues that gave me the most thought.

Out-of-hours and Evening Surgeries

Although the arrangements in Europe are broadly similar to the UK, GPs here are lucky that they are not obliged to take part in the rotas or, if under the age of fifty-five, to do nights.

I was interested in the idea, in some countries such as Sweden and Cyprus, that primary care is not necessary during the night. It is worth considering this. We have A&E departments, walk-in centres and NHS Direct. Do we need primary care facilities in the guise of co-ops as well? Are they cost-effective during the night?

Ordinary Work Day

In Cyprus the doctor starts at seven thirty in the morning and finishes at two thirty in the afternoon. In some countries the doctors, rather than doing morning and evening surgery, prefer to work from early morning to early afternoon on some days, while on others they come in about lunchtime and work until the end of the day. Is it helpful to our patients that we continue the tradition of mostly doing surgeries twice a day? Would it not be equally satisfactory in group practices if doctors did the same number of hours but did one long shift, some early and others late?

Access

As a trainer, course vocational training organiser, GP tutor and Clinical Governance lead for many years, I visited many practices and found a great variation in the ability to provide appointments. This variation was larger than the list sizes. Some doctors had no problems offering appointments within a day, while others could do no better than about two weeks. It was never clear to me what caused these differences. Advanced Access has helped in those practices that had long waiting lists but that has caused its own problems which may prove to be unacceptable. See *Private General Practice* below.

Almost every doctor I visited abroad was able to offer appointments the same day, even where, as was often the case, the list sizes were the same as ours. In addition to this, I noted that in many countries, appointments were longer than our norm of ten minutes. This was the case even when general practice was free at the time to the patients, as in Estonia, where the appointment time was twenty minutes in the practice I saw. As in the UK, I have no explanation for this phenomenon.

Range of Work

As we have seen in some countries, primary care gynaecology is done by primary care gynaecologists rather than GPs, who never do pelvic examinations. Personally, I do not see this as an advantage to patients or doctors but the system causes the creation of an extra breed of primary care specialists.

In almost all countries, cervical smears were taken by doctors, either GPs or gynaecologists, but in one country they were taken by attached midwives, if not done by gynaecologists, and in another by laboratory staff.

There is also, in many countries, another group of primary care doctors, the paediatricians. In these countries, practice varied from those where it was normal for children to be looked after by paediatricians to agreed ages, to those where the GP would often look after all children but had the right to choose not to register babies until they had reached an age where he was confident to manage them.

Because of vocational training, most British GPs are competent to do primary care gynaecology and paediatrics, and, I believe, mostly we prefer our arrangements of being responsible for these ourselves. However, speaking only for myself, I often felt uncomfortable managing ill infants. I was frightened that I would miss something vital leading to catastrophe. In fact, like most GPs, as I became more experienced, I realized I was able to recognize danger but I have seen other GPs lose this ability. Life would have been easier for me if I could have passed the responsibility for small children to the care of primary care paediatricians. Perhaps it would be worth debating the idea that GPs should have the right to refuse to register infants and alternative arrangements be made for them.

Records

The range of paperless records was similar to the UK, with most doctors on the way to becoming paperless and a few not having started.

Only in some countries did the records follow the patient; the UK is unique in having them pass through a central authority so that GPs hold life long records for most of their patients.

Although in some systems, the records were passed to the next doctor, assuming he requested them, in some the new doctor did not expect the notes and had to rely on what, if anything, the patient possessed, and often this meant starting from scratch.

I wonder how expensive it is to maintain the comprehensive and life-long records of which we are so proud. What would be lost if only a current record containing a problem list, results of all investigations and a table of medication was passed to the next doctor? This could be done by giving the patient a paper print-out or sending it to the next doctor electronically. Although I am not really advocating this, I have noticed that it seems to be satisfactory abroad and the idea is worth considering.

As well as looking after every aspect of patients' health life-long, we act as the librarian for all their medical records. As far as I know, this state of affairs has always been seen to be good and has not been questioned. On the face of it, the benefits of a complete set of records seems obvious, but could there be disadvantages? See below under *Private General Practice* and again under *Restriction of Patients.*

It was not the system in every country for consultants to report back to GPs, so records were not always complete.

Private General Practice

Certainly in Finland, and maybe other countries (unfortunately this point came up late in the tour), patients have the same rights to state funding of their prescriptions whether they see the state or private GPs. This encourages a dual system which is clearly of great benefit to patients. The most obvious advantage of this is that they can see a doctor during the day near their work, rather than as in the UK, when, if they commute, they are likely to lose half a day in order to see their GP. Other advantages are the certainty of seeing the same doctor, and frequently longer consultations.

` The disadvantages are that the private and state doctors do not communicate, so it must be difficult to know who has done what in the way of investigations and trying different treatments, and who maintains responsibility. Obviously this dual system would be political dynamite in the UK, so it is hardly worth discussing, but the practical advantages do seem worthwhile.

There is no doubt we have failed to solve the problem of access for patients who work some distance from home and it looks as though there is no solution in sight. As it is politically anathema in Britain for patients to be encouraged to have private and National Health doctors, it is going to be essential to allow people to see NHS GPs near their work who will report to their home doctors.

Restriction of Patients

We have always taken it for granted that British GPs should 'own' their patients. This is a way of saying that patients must not have any medical attention from any other doctor except in an emergency. Every medical occurrence must be reported to the GP. This makes sure that the GP is able to have a complete set of records.

I discovered that some doctors in Europe think our rules are too restrictive and mostly it is taken for granted that patients should, for example, have the right to refer themselves to private consultants without insurance penalties for the former and ethical issues for the latter. They see the benefits of this freedom, combined with the freedom of patients to go to private doctors, so great that they override the importance of the usual GP being in control and having a record of everything.

Although, as a GP, I would find it difficult to manage a patient's illnesses while there was a risk of their being investigated and treated unknown to me elsewhere, I am learning that there are two sides to this and the matter would benefit from some discussion.

Ancillary Staff and Loneliness

This is a major area and one where I realized how well-off we are in this country. Although many countries had well-staffed practices, none came to the level of the UK, where we seem to be the only country in Europe where doctors have practice managers, and almost the only one employing secretaries.

Some countries such as Austria, and Luxembourg (where they are not allowed), did not have practice nurses. The duties of nurses varied, as one would expect, but it was strange to see that some, while doing phlebotomy, were not allowed to give any form of injection. In some countries, HCAs were used instead of nurses.

The extreme, such as in Belgium, Luxembourg and France, was where the doctor worked entirely alone, from small premises or home with not even a receptionist.

I was struck by how lonely single-handed doctors seemed to be, especially if they had little or no staff either.

It was odd seeing no one between a doctor and his telephone in Belgium, and, in Austria, a single-handed doctor on her own after the last patient, backing up her computer and locking up. It is not quite the same in single-handed practices in the UK, because here the doctors at least have some staff, including their own nurses and practice managers.

Relationships with Secondary Care

The status of general practice usually seemed to be to be on a par with consultants, although, as we have seen there were exceptions, such as in Malta, Cyprus and Lithuania.

Although waiting lists varied for secondary care, I have the impression that mostly they were significantly shorter in the EU than in England.

Training

While there is training for general practice in most countries, it is done more vigorously in some than others. It appears that in the UK, it is the most stringent. We are the only country to combine the need for trainers to be visited in their practices before selection and regular re-selection. We have compulsory trainers' workshops and all the trainees have a full range of hospital-based learning for general practice, and at least a year working in one or more practices with a selected and trained trainer. All trainees must pass an examination at the end of their training before they are given a certificate which allows them to do any unsupervised work as a General Practitioner.

Quality of Life for Patients

I would like to discuss this in two parts, which I call the 'revealed' and the 'occult'.

The **revealed** part is the services the patient can see he gets, and in my opinion it is usually better everywhere than here. This is mainly because there are generally no problems with access and this is an important consideration for people, and something we have not been able to achieve here. People value the freedom to choose when to see a national health or private GP, so that they can have an appointment either near their home or place of work. They usually have the right to refer themselves to a private specialist without seeking an inaccessible GP's permission.

More contentiously in many countries, what is done by nurses here is done by the doctors there and it is thought, by the doctors anyway, that this gives them a closer relationship. Although I am told that patients would be frightened to have procedures done by nurses, especially immunisations to their children, I do not believe this is something to admire, as there seems to have been no problem in Britain building up patients' confidence in nurses.

Obviously, where the doctors are single-handed or in small groups, there is a better continuity of care than in the British large group training practices.

Practice organisation can be more patient-centred abroad. For example, as I have stated more than once, nurses who could do phlebotomy would not send patients to a laboratory for this because of lack of time themselves.

The **occult** part of quality of life for patients is more important, but needs some explaining. People do not normally know if they have high blood pressure, raised cholesterol, symptom-free diabetes or impaired glucose tolerance (which, if not addressed vigorously, is well on the way to developing diabetes), so they do not care if they are identified and treated. Although chronic disease was often identified and managed to high standards using international guidelines, this was variable and even in the best countries, apart from Holland, there were no targets or audits, let alone substantial financial incentives. It seems, therefore, that our identification and treatment of chronic disease is the best in Europe, although to be certain, we would need to demonstrate that illness and death rates from cardiovascular disease are falling faster. This would mean that there are increasingly fewer deaths from heart disease, high blood pressure and diabetes and fewer heart attacks and strokes. If this is the case, living longer and more healthily must be an enormous step in improvement in the quality of life, even if not obvious to the patients at the point of delivery. The QOF targets (discussed in *Money Matters* above) have been in place only since 2004, so, unfortunately, it is too early yet for a beneficial effect to be demonstrated. There is, however, some evidence that the number of cases of heart disease and stroke is falling faster now than the EU average.

The conflict of the revealed and the occult in the quality of care seems to me to be summarised by the patient's agenda versus the doctor's agenda. The former, what we are taught in vocational training, is what we should concentrate on and it is clearly what patients want, but it is the latter which will preserve more health and save lives. This massive problem is beautifully worded by Dr Julian Tudor Hart, a GP working in the Welsh valleys, who proved that the sort of screening I have described did, indeed, save lives. His terms are to me, apt, in that he calls the patients' agenda 'demand-led' and the doctors' screening agenda 'anticipatory care', and he had the skill to do both together. To most of us, however, this paradox is indeed the doctors' dilemma.

227

Quality of Life for Doctors

This is the place to court controversy and state that, unequivocally, life for doctors is better here than anywhere else in Europe. There are many factors which cause me to say this.

Firstly, and this is difficult, I had the impression that the income of GPs in this country is higher than elsewhere. Incomes varied throughout Europe; for example, it appears to be much higher in Italy than Spain, and where fees are paid for item of service these varied enormously. However, I could not relate this to the cost of living. Certainly the homes I visited were comfortable, but I could not adjust my mind for the spouses' income, which was unknown to me. In spite of this lack of clear evidence, I did have the feeling that we are at the top end of the scale.

Apart from our living standards, there are our working conditions. The big pluses here are our premises, staff and general lack of isolation. As I have said more than once in this work, we have secretaries and practice managers, and these are almost unknown in primary care on the continent. Where we have computers, we have clerks to back them up and often to repeat the prescriptions. The systems of practice nurses varied, but in many countries the practice nurses were more restricted in what they could do than here and, as described, often had to double up as receptionists. We see them here as very much part of our teams and they will usually attend practice clinical meetings and help us develop our protocols.

In short, we are accustomed to working in a Primary Health Care Team, a concept that is rare elsewhere.

In some countries, such as Portugal, Cyprus and Finland, the doctors are salaried and the premises are provided. In the remainder, where doctors own their practices and run them as businesses, as we do, they have to provide their own premises with little or no help from the state systems.

Other benefits of working in the UK are the lack of an assortment of annoying restrictions that are in place elsewhere. For example, there is no requirement here to take part in an out-of-hours rota and certainly no rule to make doctors younger than fifty-five work during the night. There is no law here, such as occurs in Slovenia, to prevent us doing pelvic examinations, or, as in Germany, where nurses are forbidden to give any injections, although they are allowed to take blood.

Obviously there are some problems here. Probably the worst is the feeling of the likelihood of being sued and the lack of trust that forces the need for chaperones. As we have seen, we pay much more for our defence societies than anywhere else in Europe.

Also, we work under considerable pressure. I have been an appraiser for the last three years and a constant theme when doctors are trying to implement a Personal Development Plan is the lack of time. This feeling did occur in some other countries, such as Slovenia, but it was not common. Many 'full-time' doctors, while working each weekday, did their session in the morning on some days and in the afternoon in others, and never the whole day. This was a common model.

The problems of micro-management by the state and the continuing reorganisations, which form such a burden to us here, are common to many parts of Europe.

What can we learn for the UK?

Firstly we need to ask a few simple questions. Do we need out-of-hours primary care services, at least after midnight? They are likely to be beneficial but they provide no continuity of care. If there are any advantages over A&E and the ambulance service, are they cost-effective?

Are we and our patients better keeping the same range of work? Would it be safer for patients if paediatrics and obstetrics and gynaecology were done by primary care specialists? A possible solution would be to confine the subjects to GPs with special training in these specialities, with evidence of keeping up-to-date. I believe this scheme would make sense if these GPs stuck to only one of these two disciplines.

Now we must look at two most difficult problems. The first concerns ownership of our patients, their records and access. Nowhere else in the EU are the patients 'owned' by their doctors, as here. Our patients can see GPs only at the practice where they are registered, regardless of where they work, can get national health prescriptions only from the same and, again, can turn only to their registered practice for referral to secondary care.

This system has certain advantages. It allows GPs to keep records of every illness, consultation and investigation, from cradle to grave. Every specialist or health professional is obliged to report every medical encounter to the patient's GP for entry into the notes. If a specialist is seeing a patient and needs to know about past investigations, he can turn to the GP if the latter has not already given the information in the referral letter. Unlike in many countries in the EU, it will be unlikely that two specialists are investigating a patient with the same illness at the same time unknown to each other and possibly to their GP. Lastly, because a GP's practice is responsible for a patient, he can, with modern records, make sure that the patient receives all necessary health promotion and systematic treatment of chronic diseases such as hypertension, heart disease, asthma and diabetes. This as an enormous advantage for the British patient.

Unfortunately we must examine and face the disadvantages. We have almost no arrangements for patients needing to see a doctor being able to do so near their place of work. In other countries, patients will have a National Health-equivalent doctor where they live, but if they work half an hour's journey from there, they can see a private doctor near their place of work. They pay only the fee and have the same reimbursements of the cost of their prescriptions as they would when they see their state doctor. Also, the private doctor can refer them to secondary care.

We would not like this because apart from the episode not getting into our records, we would be aware of the risk of duplicating investigations and medication trials. Perhaps we could develop a system (without necessarily waiting for the new national computer) where the private doctor is obliged to inform the National Health doctor of details of the encounter.

Only in the UK are patients so restricted that they can never see specialists without the permission of their GP. It must make business sense, if nothing else, to insist that patients using secondary care services must be referred by GPs, acting as a gatekeeper to national health clinics or hospitals. But the need for referral when a patient, however mistakenly, wishes to see a specialist privately seems to interfere with their rights. Patients with private insurance are likely to be working and find it the most difficult to get to their GP during consulting hours. Admittedly, to allow these rights leads again to problems of duplication of investigations and medication, so patients should be advised of the dangers and specialists should try to liaise with the person's GP.

The second problem is the conflict between patients' and doctors' agendas, alluded to above. I would like to explain these a little. The patient's agenda is what he wants to discuss when he makes the appointment. Some of the material may be subconscious. For the doctor to make good use of the patient's agenda he has to be skilled in listening. Take, for example, the case of a forty year old man who rarely attends, but is now complaining of chest pain. The doctor listens and thinks the symptoms are unlikely to be due to physical disease, but decides that there is just a possibility that the symptoms could be associated with heart disease, so he makes a mental note that he must examine and possibly investigate the heart to be certain nothing is being missed there. He continues to listen and hears that the patient's father died last year from lung cancer and the patient is anxious that he might be suffering from the same condition. The doctor then realises that, although he must exclude heart disease, the consultation will have failed if he does not deal with the fears about the lung cancer and make sure all is done to reassure the patient on this point. While the doctor continues to listen, he is aware that this patient does not lightly come to the surgery and so he wonders if issues of lung cancer and his father's illness and death are the main problem, so looks out for cues that might indicate other areas where the patient may be under stress.

Ever since I was a medical student, there have been debates as to whether medicine is an art or a science. To me, there has never been any doubt that medicine must be a science and anything non-scientific can normally be left to charlatans. However, the ability to listen to a patient during a consultation is the nearest that medicine gets to an art, and general practitioners are rightly proud of this skill. It is one of the most important subjects taught in vocational training and every possible point is analysed by the trainer, often using a video-recording.

The doctor's agenda, while important, is rather different. Let us assume that a sixty year old woman is coming for a routine check up for her high blood pressure. She is also suffering from headaches, due to stress and not her physical condition. She wants to use the consultation to get help for these as well as her review. In the ten minute appointment the doctor must measure the blood pressure; three times if it is raised, and average the last two readings; record the weight and write forms for various routine blood tests, which will include kidney function and cholesterol. If the blood pressure is not satisfactory he needs to discuss altering the medication and there may be a need to plead with the patient to stop smoking, and complete a form for her to attend a smoking cessation clinic, lose weight and take more exercise. It is obvious that when all this is done the headaches will get short shrift.

To sum up, in the UK we probably save more lives by having an excellent system of detecting and managing chronic disease in primary care, but it operates at the expense of depriving patients of reasonable freedoms of choice and a hopeless system of access, combined with little time to listen to our patients' needs. I believe we should try, therefore, to improve our already excellent system of general practice by examining and incorporating into our National Health Service those elements of European methods and systems which work better than ours.

Appendix

EUROPEAN GENERAL PRACTICE PROJECT
DRAFT INTERVIEW GUIDE

A. Greetings

1) Thanks for your time and trouble in your seeing me
2) Promise of confidentiality
3) I'm trying to understand what is **typical** in your country, and so if your practice is unusual in any respect please let me know
4) Before we begin the interview, please could you tell me a little about yourself and your practice, for example,
   (i)   How long have you been in practice?
   (ii) Do you work alone or in a group practice?
   (iii) How many patients do you look after?
5) How are you paid and do patients pay?

B. Problems of General Practice

1) ACCESS
   (i)   How do patients make an appointment? How long do they typically wait to get one?
   (ii) How long do you normally spend with them?
   (iii) Follow up appointments
   (iv) DNAs

(v) Are you interrupted by the phone apart from emergencies?
(vi) Do you have arrangements for telephone appointments?
(vii)Do you make house calls?

2) REFERRALS
   (i)   How easy are they? Can patients self refer?
   (ii) How long for a dermatological appointment in your system?
   (iii) How long to get a hip replacement?
   (iv) Cataracts?

3) CONTINUITY OF CARE
   Are patients attached to their practice at any one time in your system?

4) RECORDS
   (i)   How do you keep records?
   (ii) Do you have templates or fields?
   (iii) Do records follow the patient?
   (iv) What computer codes do you use?

5) INVESTIGATIONS

6) PRESCRIBING
   (i)   Do you have a system for repeat prescribing?
   (ii) Do you have any practice guidelines for prescribing?
   (iii) Is a consultation expected to finish with a prescription?
   (iv) Are you free to prescribe what you think best or are there financial constraints? Are you encouraged in generic prescribing and if so what percentage have you reached? What are your views about this?

7) HEALTH PROMOTION

8) STAFF
Do you have practice nurses and what do they do for you? What other staff do you have?

9) RANGE OF WORK.
   (i) Do patients come to you for O&G and childcare?
   (ii) What are the arrangements for immunisation?

10) INTERNET ACCESS

11) DEPRESSION

12) CERTIFICATES

13) ALTERNATIVE MEDICINE

C. Educational development and standards

1) Do you have local or national guidelines for treatment?
   (i) Chronic disease such as IHD, hypertension, diabetes and asthma? How many of these illnesses are treated in primary care?
   (ii) Do you have a smoking cessation policy?
   (iii) Use of antibiotics? And treatment of sore throat.

2) What are the arrangements for continuing medical education?
3) Are you encouraged to have a Personal Development Plan?
4) Do you have Significant Event discussions?
5) Do you have any sort of appraisal?
6) Do you have any form of reaccreditation?
7) Are GPs monitored in any way? If so, in what way and by whom? Are there any procedures in place to deal with poorly performing GPs or practices?

D. Vocational Training

E. Out-of-hours Care

Printed in the United States
216160BV00003B/13/P